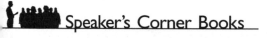

Speaker's Corner Books

is a provocative new series designed to stimulate, educate, and foster discussion on significant public policy topics. Written by experts in a variety of fields, these brief and engaging books should be read by anyone interested in the trends and issues that shape our society.

More thought-provoking titles
in the Speaker's Corner series

The Brave New World of Health Care
  Richard D. Lamm

The Enduring Wilderness:
Protecting Our Natural Heritage through the Wilderness Act
  Doug Scott

Ethics for a Finite World:
An Essay Concerning a Sustainable Future
  Herschel Elliott

God and Caesar in America:
An Essay on Religion and Politics
  Gary Hart

One Nation Under Guns:
An Essay on an American Epidemic
  Arnold Grossman

On the "Clean" Road Again:
Biodiesel and the Future of the Family Farm
  Willie Nelson

Parting Shots from My Brittle Bow:
Reflections on American Politics and Life
  Eugene J. McCarthy

Red Alert!:
Saving the Planet with Indigenous Knowledge
Daniel R. Wildcat

Social Security and the Golden Age:
An Essay on the New American Demographic
George McGovern

TABOR and Direct Democracy:
An Essay on the End of the Republic
Bradley J. Young

Think for Yourself!:
An Essay on Cutting through the Babble, the Bias, and the Hype
Steve Hindes

Two Wands, One Nation:
An Essay on Race and Community in America
Richard D. Lamm

For more information, visit our Web site,
www.fulcrumbooks.com

Condition Critical

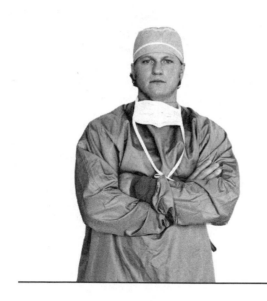

Condition Critical

A New Moral Vision for Health Care

Richard D. Lamm
and Robert H. Blank

Condition Critical

A New Moral Vision for Health Care

Richard D. Lamm
and Robert H. Blank

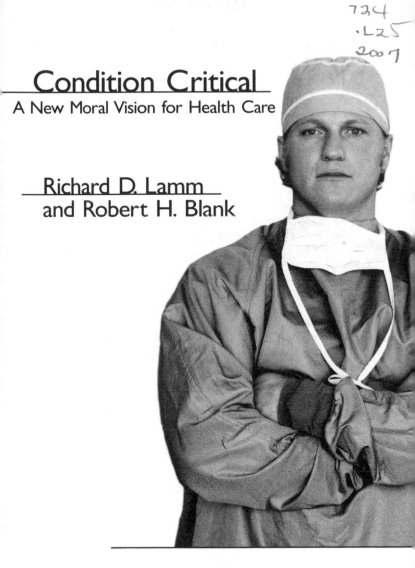

 Fulcrum Publishing

Golden, Colorado

© 2007 Richard D. Lamm and Robert H. Blank

Library of Congress Cataloging-in-Publication Data

Lamm, Richard D.
  Condition critical : a new moral vision for health care / Richard D. Lamm and Robert H. Blank.
    p. ; cm. -- (Speaker's corner books)
  Includes bibliographical references.
  ISBN-13: 978-1-55591-612-1
  ISBN-10: 1-55591-612-0
  1. Medical ethics. 2. Medical technology--Moral and ethical aspects. 3. Health care rationing. 4. Medical policy. I. Blank, Robert H. II. Title. III. Series.
  [DNLM: 1. Health Care Rationing--ethics--United States. 2. Attitude to Health--United States. 3. Ethical Relativism--United States. 4. Health Care Rationing--trends--United States. 5. Health Care Reform--trends--United States. WA 540 AA1 L232c 2007]
  R724.C6647 2007
  362.1--dc22
                              2006101595

Printed in Canada by Friesens Corporation
0 9 8 7 6 5 4 3 2 1

Design: Jack Lenzo
Editorial: Sam Scinta, Faith Marcovecchio
Cover image: © 2006 Index Open

Fulcrum Publishing
4690 Table Mountain Drive, Suite 100
Golden, Colorado 80403
800-992-2908 • 303-277-1623
www.fulcrumbooks.com

Contents

Preface

This book is meant to wake America up to a coming public-policy train wreck. Three seemingly unstoppable trends in America are on a collision course: (1) the inventiveness of the promoters of medical technology, (2) health care provider's allegiance to the Hippocratic oath, and (3) the health care expectations of the American public. America is sleeping as this collision draws nearer. As Winston Churchill warned us seventy years ago, democracies always seem to wake up twenty years too late. Yet even if America awoke tomorrow, it would be too late to avoid many aspects of the coming collision. A related but compounding factor is that though we must adopt new and unpopular policies in health care, we must do so simultaneously as we fix Social Security and provide comprehensive long-term care. As the baby boomers retire, all three challenges of an aging society must be considered together.

Two major transforming realities have overtaken the health care system in the last thirty years that require America to develop a new moral vision: (1) taxpayers now fund approximately 50 percent of health care, and (2) it is now inescapably clear that resources are limited relative to needs. When limited funds and resources meet unlimited demands, budgets must be imposed and priorities made. When this occurs, the rationing of health care goes from outrage to obligation, from intolerable to inescapable. Those who distribute pooled or taxpayer funds become not mere payment agents but the allocators of limited resources who must maximize the health of the group they cover. Though it seems counterintuitive, there can be better health through rationing. A thoughtful distribution of limited resources produces more health than indiscriminately throwing money at health care.

This book will be controversial. Some of the decisions America will have to make will make our moral compasses spin. As the avalanche of baby boomers hits retirement age and their high-cost health care years, America will be forced to make a series of choices that we have no tradition in making. America has been great at distributing the bounty of a growing continent, but it has had little practice reducing benefits and expectations. We have built a system without brakes, where "can do" has become "must do" and the threat of lawsuits hangs over the whole system like a Sword of Damocles. This system is unsustainable, and large-scale changes will need to take place. Our situation is similar to the negotiation of a union contract: the most difficult aspect of union negotiations is when a company must ask for *take-backs*, i.e., when it has to take back benefits previously given. America is going to have to take back health care on a massive scale.

> Simply put, medical science has invested, discovered, and ethically self-imposed more medical care than those who pay for it can afford.

Simply put, medical science has invested, discovered, and ethically self-imposed more medical care than those who pay for it can afford. Medicare and Medicaid, as we know them, are unsustainable. These are land mines in our children's future. No modern nation can afford to do everything the Hippocratic oath requires for all its citizens. The explosion of technology and our aging society demands we rethink the meaning and scope of this ancient oath.

Two of the basic foundations of American health care—that a patient has a right to expect any and all medicine that is wanted or beneficial to his or her health and that a doctor has the right to prescribe and deliver all the health care he or she feels is appropriate—need to be challenged, and that must begin with a look at the doctor-patient relationship. In health care, nothing is more important than patient and physician autonomy. It is the Golden Rule of Medicine. But new economic realities are changing that Golden Rule. Current health care spending is unsustainable. No physician and no patient can expect a blank check when there are other parties involved, those who pay 83 percent of American health care: private insurers and the government.

Currently, the solutions to the real problems of health care are hardly being talked or written about. Neither political party begins to have a solution to the health care problem equal to its magnitude. Few scholars have seriously considered what really has to be done to moderate this escalation of health care spending. It will require a change in medical practice, medical ethics, health care culture, but, most important of all, the expectations of the American public. Moreover, these changes will involve new trade-offs heretofore thought unimaginable: trade-offs between quality of life and quantity of life, young versus old, acute medicine versus preventive medicine, and health care versus everything else the government funds. These problems are exacerbated by the state of the U.S.

economy, which is likely heading for some rough times that will further compound the problems raised here. It is apparent that all the economic indicators are bad for the future: Americans' negative savings rate, the government borrowing $2 billion a day from countries abroad to maintain our current consumption patterns, and our twin deficits, the federal deficit and the trade deficit. On the other hand, this could be a time of great opportunity for new ideas such as those presented here, which may be the galvanizing event we need to reform health care. We are approaching a time when change will be inevitable and inescapable.

Chapter 1

A New Moral Vision

> *The choices we face are clear and painful. The United States can suffer a continual increase in medical expenditures yielding benefits worth less than costs. Or it can impose effective limits. If it follows the second course, it will have to confront a long list of decisions on which discussion has not begun.*
> —Henry J. Aaron and William B. Schwartz,
> The Painful Prescription

No modern nation can build a health care system a patient at a time. No citizen can expect, in this time of technological marvels, all the health care that modern medicine can provide. No physician can practice his or her profession assuming he or she is the unrestrained advocate of every patient. No citizen can expect and no nation can afford to give the Hippocratic oath a blank check. Modern medicine is awash in twenty-first-century technology guided by twentieth- and even nineteenth-century thinking. Nothing in the past history of American health care has prepared us for the new decisions and dilemmas that we face. The longer we wait, the more difficult the problem will become. There is no way within the existing dialogue or thinking to solve America's problem of runaway costs in health care. We are sailing uncharted waters.

Our current medical culture and practice, aggravated by unrealistic citizen expectations, is misallocating hundreds of billions of dollars, which the nation cannot afford and which is leaving a crushing burden on our children and grandchildren. We spend more money than any other nation on health care but rank poorly on comparative measures of health. There are third-world countries with a per capita income one-twentieth of ours that keep their citizens, in many respects, as healthy or healthier than Americans. We have a technologically superb but socially inadequate and administratively inefficient health care system. New thinking, not new technology, is our most immediate need. We need a new moral vision for American health care.

> There are third-world countries with a per capita income one-twentieth of ours that keep their citizens, in many respects, as healthy or healthier than Americans.

This new moral vision must look beyond the individual patient-doctor relationship and develop new roles for the individual, third-party payers, and the state and nation. A new moral landscape must be devised that adds new actors to the historic physician-patient relationship. Medical ethics, physician autonomy, and citizen expectations all grew out of a time when there was not that much that could be done for a patient. A physician today, with the stroke of a pen, can cause more medicine to be delivered to a patient than most physicians in the past could spend in a professional lifetime. The hand that once held a simple black bag now commands medical technology that can bankrupt a hospital for a single patient. Health care is a fiscal black hole into which we can pour literally all the nation's wealth.

Health care has been growing for the last fifty years at over twice the rate of inflation. No item of any budget can grow at over twice the rate of inflation. Health care already receives one out of every seven dollars spent in America. For all its technological miracles, for all its dedication and caring, modern American medicine is unsustainable and will soon be unaffordable. In a world of international economic competition, our goods and services contain twice the health care costs of the goods and services of our international competitors. Modern medicine, driven by a culture of caring and haunted by the shadow of a lawsuit, can make our nation economically sick. For the health of the nation, and to maximize the health of its citizens, we need to rethink modern health care.

The Next New Deal

The New Deal, with its many social programs, including those that addressed the health of our citizens, was so mesmerizing to a generation of public-policy makers, so just, so right for the time, so politically stabilizing, that it has dominated our thinking for sixty-five years. It deserves to have done so, because the more we look at the Depression in hindsight, the more we recognize how prescient the New Deal was, how large the stakes, how appropriate the response. But many of these institutions are demographically obsolete. We are living too long and having too few children to continue them without substantial amendment. Today, 83 percent of American health care is raised collectively through either government or insurance. Medicare and Medicaid are forty years old and Social Security is seventy years old, and neither serves the interest of the younger generations that increasingly fund them. We must see pragmatically and address without nostalgia the new circumstances with which we are faced. We must rethink, reevaluate, and reconceptualize old programs to meet a new era.

Modernizing the New Deal will be much more difficult than initiating it was, because of the popularity of the programs. Both political parties vocally support Social Security and Medicare and have a large stake politically in making the right decisions concerning them. They are among the most popular governmental programs in America. The sheer weight of a popular success and the drag of the status quo compound the magnitude of what faces us, and it is understandable why many people do not want to substantially amend this system. To admit that our system of funding health care through existing public and private programs is unsustainable requires us to give up the dream of a totally universal and egalitarian health care system. To many people, this is the death of a dream. Like take-backs in the union movement, it is unacceptable to many people that we should give back benefits painfully achieved, no matter what the facts dictate.

This means we will need leadership—strong bipartisan leadership that until now has been lacking. The public is already distrustful of the political process, and individual citizens are wrapped up in their own needs and lives. With the nation now politically divided almost equally, it will be hard to prepare the public for the type and magnitude of change necessary. How does a democracy downsize expectations? How do we make the unpalatable at least digestible?

Goethe warned, "If we are going to live in our father's

house, we must rebuild it." Every generation must rethink and readapt the institutions they inherit to the new realities they face. Our task as Americans, however difficult, must be to rebuild the house of health care. We have overbuilt and overfurnished the doctor-patient floor and amassed an imposing economic configuration, and there are high stakes in its perpetuation. But most of the rest of the structure remains not only unfinished, but also unframed.

There is more than one level, or "floor," in health policy: legislators, health plans, and family members have different moral duties than doctors, and we need different levels of ethical analysis for each, corresponding to the competing levels of moral obligation. Moreover, health policy is not an island, complete in itself, but is instead part of the landscape of many needs.

> Health policy is not an island, complete in itself, but is instead part of the landscape of many needs.

Our aging society has three overriding public-policy issues if it is to have a just and adequate system. It must provide health care, income security, and long-term care, and we must be wise enough to balance the spending among not only these needs, but while also meeting the full spectrum of other governmental demands. It is a big task. But instead of leading to despair, the problems raised here should be viewed as a challenge: to fashion a fundamentally more equitable and sustainable health care system, one that addresses the moral needs at all levels, not just the one. This is a challenge to use the same sort of ingenuity that gave us the New Deal. Without a broadened vision along these lines, the outlook for future generations will be ominous. We must find within our generation some of the same courage, creativity, and prescience that inspired the New Deal generation.

Seeing the Big Picture: An Expanded Moral Vision

Proust once observed that "The real voyage of discovery is not seeking new lands but seeing with new eyes." The same could be said of our view of the current health care situation in America: We must look at its new demographic realities with new eyes. We must look fully and honestly at what it means to run a nation of fifty Floridas, where every state is largely composed of an elderly population. Doing so is troubling to us because it challenges long-held assumptions of unlimited resources and ever-heightened standards of living. It is especially disconcerting in the United States' individualistic-centered culture because it requires addressing collective societal interests at the perceived expense of individuals. Thus our need to see the world, as Proust suggests, with new eyes.

To help us in that process, it is useful to recognize that a new moral vision for health care is built on distinct moral duties at each of three levels of health care, duties that at times are in competition with each other. These levels are (1) the individual patient in the doctor-patient relationship, (2) the third-party payer, and (3) the state and/or nation. Each of these levels in health policy has a different moral radius; in other words, each has distinct though overlapping moral roles.

In order to address the problems facing health policy, we must examine each level of health care and how that level interacts and overlaps with the others and then construct a coherent method of analysis. All levels owe a duty to the individual patient, but not the same duty. The moral radius of a physician is almost entirely to his or her patient; the moral radius of the insurance company or group has a duty mostly to its subscribers; whereas the state and nation has a duty to all its citizens—for government, its geographic jurisdiction becomes its moral jurisdiction.

The Individual Patient

The foundation of all health, and consequently health care, is the individual. We have a duty, and the means, to provide all citizens with a comprehensive package of preventive services and primary care as well as long-term rehabilitative and mental health services. But to accomplish this without national bankruptcy, we must put some new responsibilities and duties on the individual.

As Americans, our biggest health threat lies within our own habits and lifestyle. Health threats used to come mostly from disease and other causes outside the individual; today, thanks to the successes of modern medicine, most of the infectious diseases are either gone or pose minimal threat. Our habits and lifestyles are much more likely to bring us to an untimely end or severe sickness. For that reason, every person's best doctor is him- or herself.

> As Americans, our biggest health threat lies within our own habits and lifestyle.

But in the current scheme of things, individuals feel that unending health care is their right, regardless of personal behavior. As imminent physician John Knowles put it, "The cost of sloth, gluttony, alcoholic intemperance, reckless driving, sexual frenzy, and smoking is now a national and not just an individual responsibility. This is justified as individual freedom—but one man's freedom in health is another man's shackle in taxes and insurance premiums. I believe the idea of a 'right' to health should be replaced by an idea of an individual moral obligation to preserve one's own health—a duty, if you will." The conventional notion of rights—including "a right to health care" excludes responsibility for personal behavior. A revised concept would shift emphasis heavily toward personal responsibility (see Chapter 3 for a full discussion of this). Under this approach, those who fail to act responsibly and protect their health would in large measure lose their claim upon societal health resources.

The individual-responsibility model is necessary because the individual alone can now avoid most diseases. Why not shift the monetary burden to those individuals who knowingly take health risks? We do not advocate abandoning a person with bad habits, but we do need heightened individual responsibility put in balance with fairness. Medical ethicist Robert Veatch said it so well: "I reach the conclusion that it is fair, that it is just, if persons in need of health services resulting from true, voluntary risks are treated differently from those in need of the same services for other reasons. In fact it would be unfair if the two groups were treated equally."

> Medical treatment that adds to the quality of our individual lives can occasionally become destructive when considered cumulatively in a society that has many other pressing needs.

Can physicians and other health providers live with this? We say yes, and Reinhardt Priester details how physicians could create such a system: "Providers should help to develop allocation rules and then play by the rules. Within those rules, they should continue to advocate zealously for their individual patient's interests. If providers believe the rules are detrimental to their patients, they should work to change them."

Allocating health care in this way has become a necessity, for, as we see in current health care practice, we can truly have "too much of a good thing." Individual "goods" can become collective "bads." Medical treatment that adds to the quality of our individual lives can occasionally become destructive when considered cumulatively in a society that has many other pressing needs. A succession of altruistic actions to individuals can, under certain circumstances, cumulatively turn into negative public policy. There is what Herschel Elliott has called a *moral reversal* at work here: beyond a certain level of effort and expenditures on an individual, ethical conduct becomes unethical excess.

Pressures emerging from the health care crisis necessitate a much closer look at the role individuals play in contributing to their own health problems, a shift of responsibility for health toward the individual, and a renewed emphasis on the obligations of individuals to society to do those things that maximize health. A major part of this effort must be aimed at reducing expectations of the public regarding the availability of health care resources; reducing individuals' unrealistic demands for curative medicine would make them personally accountable for their individual actions. Americans must realize the necessity for limits and end the fatuous assumption of unlimited resources perpetuated in a consumptive society.

> Americans must realize the necessity for limits and end the fatuous assumption of unlimited resources perpetuated in a consumptive society.

The Doctor-Patient Relationship

For 2,000 years, physicians have been patient advocates. A caring physician was, at one time, the only constant weapon in our medical arsenal. When a physician couldn't cure (which was often), he could at least care. This 2,000-year-old tradition stresses the role of the physician as advocate, fiduciary, healer, and confidant of the patient. This role remains the foundation of health care worldwide. Yet however important this foundation is, modern medicine cannot stop there. A patient advocate spending pooled money does not make the best distributor of limited resources. Providers do not realize how many alternate uses there are for the money they freely spend. They are focused on their patients, and that should remain their focus. For though physicians may be the most important single actor in health care, it is third-party payers that now fund most of U.S. health care. Those third-party payers are themselves moral agents with their own moral duties. They have an independent duty to use the resources under their control wisely and to maximize the health of those they fund. They must do more than blindly pay the bills, as we will explore below.

American physicians think of third-party payers as intruders (a term borrowed from philosopher Haavi Morreim) who too often question their judgments, but inevitably they must be thought of as partners in the health transaction. The only way third-party payers can morally discharge their duties as trustees of limited resources is to set priorities and strategies for maximizing the money under their control. No pool of resources can be raised from cost-conscious buyers and spent by health-conscious patients and their passionate advocates without a mechanism for limits. If we didn't have parsimonious third-party payers, we would have to invent them. If we remove the profit motive, everything a third-party payer does prevents it from doing something else to advance the health of the group. The price of allocating limited funds is the painful necessity to determine limits, make trade-offs, and set priorities.

Once we honestly admit that health care is not an

open-ended system, the whole dialogue changes. As David Eddy notes:

> The acid test for whether financial resources are limited is to simply ask those who are responsible for budgets of health plans whether they have enough money to do everything everyone wants to do. If not, then the budget is limited. We will need to accept, once and for all, that resources are limited. It is the limitation on resources that both necessitates and justifies the strategy of getting more for less.

Once we face up to the reality of making unlimited demands fit limited resources, the physician's obligations must be synchronized with that of the funder. Increasingly, health policy analysts such as Peter Ubel are recognizing that this will require a change in the total advocacy of the physician for the patient: "Health care rationing will succeed only if physicians relax their advocacy duties occasionally (cautiously and carefully) to ration at the bedside."

Ubel argues that if someone has to set limits, better to have the physician involved in the process rather than excluded from it. Haavi Morreim makes a similar argument. She points out that given all the interventions modern medicine can bring to an aging population, health care is simply going to learn to live, every day and every way, with fiscal scarcity. Unlike past rationing, which was rare and isolated, these cost-conscious pressures will be ubiquitous and even more morally troubling: "It is one thing to refuse an item because there is none of it available, and quite another to say that even though it is available, it will not be used because of its expense." But making a virtue out of necessity, she states, "Fiscal scarcity ... requires us to examine more carefully the legitimate competing claims of society, of payers, of other patients, and of other providers for the health care system's limited resources." Howard Hiatt makes a related point in his classic article "Protecting the Medical Commons" when he argues that physicians must play an integral part in determining the rationing polices and priorities, for, however burdensome, no other entity can begin to do it as well. Physicians cannot stand back and have others make these decisions or they will essentially lose their clinical authority.

The historic geniuses of medicine have had an almost consuming focus on the patient. But professions, like individuals, often find that their strengths are also their weaknesses. The health of a nation is much more than 600,000 physicians treating 300 million patients. The total focus on the patient, which served us well for a time, is outdated, unaffordable, and obsolete. It has become, when applied to an entire population, an economic cancer. No doctor can send, and no patient can expect, unlimited resources.

> Physicians must play an integral part in determining the rationing polices and priorities, for, however burdensome, no other entity can begin to do it as well.

Thus in a world of limited resources, both health plans and public policy must inevitably suboptimize the publicly funded health care delivered to the individual so as to maximize the health of the group or society. This means that physicians will have to cooperate with these new moral actors, even if it means giving up some of their traditional autonomy.

The Third-Party Payer

Let us role-play. Assume you are the medical director of a health insurance company. What would you consider the scope of your moral obligations? Clearly, in this day and age, it cannot be to simply pay all claims that doctors (and other providers) submit for those insured by you. Yes, you check for fraud and excess billing, but do you not have an independent obligation to maximize the health of all those you insure? We cannot simultaneously optimize the health of each individual insured and also maximize the health of the total group; there is often a conflict between the two. As Haavi Morreim explains, "Our traditionally narrow focus must now be explicitly complemented with other notions of justice." We need a new concept of justice for both those who allocate resources for a group and for those who belong to that group. Morreim calls this *contributive justice* and points out that when one is in a group of insured people, one person's excess takes away resources that are needed by others in the group.

One of the greatest prospects for American public policy to increase the health of the nation is to differentiate between the macroallocation and the microallocation of resources. Those who distribute commonly collected resources (tax monies and health premiums) among a group of people macroallocate. Health providers microallocate when they focus on decisions regarding particular patients. We must better think through these two roles because, as Frank Lewins points out, "The distinction between macroallocation and microallocation of resources is crucial. More traditional bioethical analysis might clarify the microallocation issues, but it is inappropriate at the macroallocation level and therefore misses the point." It misses the point because the individual focus of biomedical ethics is too narrow to be useful in the macroallocation by payers. Macroallocation involves trade-offs and setting priorities. Existing biomedical ethics have been developed, as have most professional codes of ethics concentrating on individual treatment. That is as it should be. But the macroallocation of resources, as Lewins points out, is "best understood as a political issue rather than an ethical issue."

Distributing commonly collected resources among a group of patients involves very different dynamics

> Those distributing commonly collected funds do not have the luxury of thinking in terms of individualized care.

than a health provider caring for patients individually does. Those distributing commonly collected funds do not have the luxury of thinking in terms of individualized care. Government must provide multiple services to its citizens, and health insurers must provide services to multiple beneficiaries. Both have more-comprehensive duties to a wider group of beneficiaries than a physician does to his patients. Therefore, the scope of the differences between macroallocation and microallocation is considerable. Simply put, they have very different jobs to do, as the figure on page 29 illustrates.

No nation, state, or health plan in the macroallocation of its funds can assume that its health care distributions meet the cumulative medical needs of all its individual members. This is clearer in other nations where the government more directly funds health care, as Rudolf Klein details:

MACROALLOCATION	MICROALLOCATION
Asks: How do you keep a society or a group healthy?	Asks: How do you keep an individual patient healthy?
Tools: Health policy, education, public safety, smoking control, system reform, etc.	Tools: Medicine and teaching healthy habits
Standards: Equal protection, due process, political pressures. Asks: What spending patterns keep the group healthy?	Standards: "Beneficial" delivery with the focus exclusively on the patient
Goal: Maximize good	Goal: Do no harm
Asks: How do we best deliver health to the group or society?	Asks: Is it good medicine?
Cost: Must always be a consideration	Cost: Not a consideration
Maximize health of the group	Maximize health of the patient
Asks: Why do people die before their time? (Smoking, alcohol abuse, poor diet, etc.)	Asks: What do people die of? (Heart disease, cancer, etc.)

This [governmental] perspective shifts the focus of resource allocation decisions from the characteristics of individuals to the characteristics of the groups to which those individuals belong. ... For if maximizing collective welfare trumps maximizing individual benefits, then it is information about the impact of specific resource allocation policies rather than information about the characteristics of individual would-be beneficiaries that becomes crucial.

We must better reconcile individual need with the common resources that fund most of that individual need. A health provider can theoretically meet all of the medical needs of its patients; a state can never meet all the health needs of all its citizens. A health provider can focus on an individual, but a government must meet many needs, both health and otherwise, for all its citizens in a world of trade-offs and priorities. Health providers ration when they fail to provide a medical service to an individual patient. A state or nation, however, rations both when it denies a needed medical benefit and also when it fails to provide universal coverage. Therefore, all governments ration medicine in one way or another. As Will Gaylin has observed, "Our nation has a health care crisis, and rationing is the only solution. There is no honorable way that we Americans can duck this responsibility."

Once we stop avoiding this responsibility, we inevitably must recognize that there is occasionally a conflict between the goal and ethics of paying for health care with commonly collected funds (macroallocation) and the goals and ethics in delivering health care (microallocation). To recognize this will be politically difficult but is socially inevitable. It will require a change in the cultural values of both citizens and health providers, but the rewards are gargantuan. America can deliver more health to its citizens for less money once it adopts a broader moral vision of health care in modern society.

The State or Nation

Let us continue to role-play. Suppose you are in the U.S. Senate, one of America's 100 politically elite. You have a passion to keep America healthy. Your patient now is the American public, and your goal is to maximize the health of 300 million Americans. Where do you begin? What questions do you ask? It is not an easy task. The responsibility is heavy and the stakes are high. You soon come face to face with a crucial problem: do you seek health for America or for 300 million Americans? You soon find that the difference is immense. If you think of your job as maximizing the health of 300 million individuals, you start down a very different road than if you feel your duty is to maximize America's health. A very different vision is needed than thinking traditionally of the sum total of 300 million individual Americans, most (not unreasonably) seeking to protect against every health hazard and each served by a doctor trained as a patient advocate to (again, not surprisingly) monomaniacally serve and protect that patient.

Our current system maximizes demand for medical services paid for with pooled resources within a system that insulates patients from the cost. People usually buy health care with free or deeply discounted dollars. No system, public or private, can allow people to consume as worried patients and fund as parsimonious taxpayers or ratepayers. Someone must judge whether or not a medical intervention is a fair and reasonable expenditure of the group's limited funds. The road that looks exclusively at individuals is ultimately a dead end. The other road asks, "How do we maximize the health of America?"

> Our current system maximizes demand for medical services paid for with pooled resources within a system that insulates patients from the cost.

This is, normally, the customary public-policy question. Public policy generally looks to populations, not individuals. It asks, for example, "How do we defend America?" not "How do we defend each and every American?" We build highways for populations, not individuals. We never build a fire department or a police department by asking how we keep *you* safe. We must inevitably ask how we keep the *community* safe. No modern government can build an adequate service system by trying to serve individual needs. It must look to serving the total community.

When we try to build public policy around the individual, we are not only doomed to failure, but we end up acting counterproductively. We run smack into the "trag-edy of the commons" problem, where every person seek-ing his or her own self-interest in a finite world ends up destroying the common resource (in this case the money we have to spend on health). To even attempt to build a health care system around individuals ironically does not (and cannot) maximize the health of the nation or its elderly. The health of the nation cannot and should not be the cumulative health needs of its individual citizens.

Doctors look at trees; public policy looks at forests. That is not a criticism. Caring for their patients a patient at a time is what medicine is all about. But it is not what health is all about. As a U.S. senator, you must ask, "How do we keep America healthy?" The individual citizen is important, but individual needs cannot be allowed to trump public needs. Keeping a nation healthy requires public-policy makers to look at the entire health land-scape. What are the nation's health hazards? Why do citizens die before their time? How do we keep the nation as healthy as possible?

> The uninsured do not belong to a phy-sician, or an insurance company, but to the government, which should clearly own the problem of ensuring every citizen good basic health care.

The first answer is to give all citizens good basic health care. Policy makers cannot continue to ignore the uninsured, because they "own" the problem of the uninsured. The uninsured do not belong to a physician, or an insurance company, but to the government, which should clearly own the problem of ensuring every citizen good basic health care.

Next in keeping a society healthy are health promo-tion and public health policies directed at things such as smoking, diet, and alcohol. Can we find strategies that save the most lives and bring the most health to the nation by reducing or eliminating these health hazards? Public money should help maximize the health and well-being of the public, before as well as after citizens become ill. The broad public concern, then, is how we spend limited resources to keep America healthy in balance with the cost of addressing citizens' other social needs. No common pool of funds collected by third-party payers can ultimately ignore the law of diminishing returns. If every American would get all the *beneficial* health care demanded by current medical ethics and practice, it would create an unethical society where medical care would crowd out too many other important social goods. Medical ethics provide no mechanism to weigh and balance individual health needs with other social or group needs. However elegantly reasoned, medical ethics cannot control the practical allocation of pooled funds.

> We are fooling ourselves when we do not admit that we ration in America. We in fact limit health care in one of the cruelest ways that any nation can limit medicine: by simply leaving people out of the system.

Once the government starts to play a role in health care, it has to prioritize needs and set limits. This is already being done in other places in the world. The method varies, but all other countries set limits better than we do. We are fooling ourselves when we do not admit that we ration in America as well. We in fact limit health care in one of the cruelest ways that any nation can limit medicine: by simply leaving people out of the system. But there are better ways of allocating limited funds. In a world of limited resources, you cannot explore their best use, the so-called opportunity costs of each dollar, unless you set priorities on what you can afford. We must start a community dialogue about how we can put our health care dollars to the highest and best use. It is an inevitable dialogue, and we ought to make a virtue out of necessity.

America finds itself in a public-policy Catch-22, where public policy historically relies on a medical culture and ethical standards that are bound to bankrupt it while at the same time allows us to ignore larger, more important funding for other, nonmedical social needs. No profession can claim public resources in isolation from other social needs. From a public-policy viewpoint, we have built the house of health care ethics on an inadequate foundation. To the extent that taxpayer monies fund our health care system, that system must prove its worth amidst all competing social needs. Our health care system must be consistent with our economic realities and the survival of other social priorities. The ethics of good medical intentions must be grounded in economic reality. Government simply cannot write into law, nor can it base a reimbursement system, on a code of ethics developed by a profession. If we take seriously the World Health Organization's comprehensive definition of health (complete physical, mental, and social well-being), public policy must consider panoramically the entire public-policy landscape. As the Canadian study *The Determinants of Health* concludes: "For more than half a century the understanding that there is much more to health than health care has been largely ignored, despite the fact that increased spending on the formal health care system is no longer having a corresponding positive impact on overall population health."

> America finds itself in a public-policy Catch-22, where public policy historically relies on a medical culture and ethical standards that are bound to bankrupt it while at the same time allows us to ignore larger, more important funding for other, nonmedical social needs.

When a state attempts to maximize health, it is not making individual moral judgments. It has a different and broader moral radius than a physician. It is allocating resources where they will do the most good. Oregon decided to ration benefits rather than ration uninsured people. The state made less high-technology medicine available, but provided basic health care to most people. It was allocating limited resources using all the relevant considerations available, trying to achieve a just and equitable Medicaid system that maximized health benefits to all Oregonians. It was an empirical process that should not be evaluated by the medical ethics of the doctor-patient relationship.

> When a state attempts to maximize health, it is not making individual moral judgments. ... It is allocating resources where they will do the most good.

A sustainable, publicly funded health care system must look beyond the individual to the justice of the system. It must step above medical ethics and ask what ethical public policy is. It cannot be content to merely fund all doctor-patient relationships, but must try to maximize the health of society using a variety of tools. It is a world of trade-offs, priority setting, and rationing. Ethical health care system must, inevitably, incorporate all three.

A related issue at the state and national level is that medical research into increasingly marginal health care is crowding out many of our other societal needs. We are developing more and more high-cost, low-benefit medical technology in a society that offers health care to fewer and fewer people at a higher and higher cost. As former National Institutes of Health director Harold Varmus observed:

We have a problem in this country in that there is nothing people place a higher value on than a healthy life, but I'm concerned about two things—the number we allocate to health becoming just too great to sustain, even for people who are relatively well to do, but more troubling is the idea that we're going to cut a very significant portion of our population out of the benefits of certain kinds of approaches to health that were paid for by public money and ought to be publicly accessible.

A basic issue that must be confronted is what proportion of our resources we are willing and able to put into these highly intensive and expensive medical interventions.

Seeing the Problem of Intergenerational Equity

One great step forward taken by the New Deal was to see clearly the plight of the elderly and poor. Today's challenge is to see what the solutions to past problems are doing to future generations. We must enlarge our concept of justice as we did for other forgotten or ignored people and interests and start to see and evaluate distributional issues in light of justice across the generations. What are the impacts of today's policies on the future of our children and grandchildren? Regardless of political party, our generation has liberally used credit. Our leaders have been elected and reelected partly by encumbering our children. However much wealth our generation has created, in public policy we have not fully paid our own way. Furthermore, we have grossly understated our governmental debt and overstated our assets. The unfunded liability we leave our children is closer to $70 trillion, when accounted correctly according to standard accounting rules, than the $8.5 trillion federal debt we admit to. In addition, we have created an ocean of contingent liabilities that may come due if the economic dominos start to fall. We have also overstated the assets we have left to cover these obligations; for instance, many claim there is no meaningful value in the Social Security Trust Fund. When a generation inherits "bonds" from the previous generation, they inherit nothing of value. The bond is offset by the inheritors' obligation to pay the bond.

We need to recognize that however successful and however popular our entitlement programs are, they have become unjust to our children who are paying into them. This applies with special urgency to our health care programs. The new but painful obligation of modern medicine is to develop systems that set goals, limits, and priorities that are consistent with total societal reform. Whoever distributes limited funds must decide generally what is worth paying for and what isn't worth paying for in light of total need. Limited funds should be budgeted according to relative need, and it is the duty of those allocating the pooled resources to set up a system of priorities that will maximize the health of the total group.

> Whoever distributes limited funds must decide generally what is worth paying for and what isn't worth paying for in light of total need.

Both public policy and health plans have the obligation to look at the opportunity costs of pooled money. They must, for instance, compare the costs of using more-expensive contrasting dyes in X-rays and scanning (and avoiding a small risk) with the possibility of saving lives in other areas, such as mammography, Pap smears, or improved cardiac care. All options to maximize limited funds should be weighed and considered. Southern

California Kaiser has shown that it can save twice as many women for two-thirds the money by concentrating mammography on women in the age group with the greatest risk. Kaiser recognized that to optimize the health of the group, you must occasionally suboptimize what is available to the individual. This bites deeply into existing practice and culture. But it must be done. The price of modern medicine is to see the inevitability and desirability of forming strategies that fit infinite demands into finite resources. The challenge of American health care, especially in our aging society, is a particularly difficult one because it involves downsizing citizens' expectations of what is to be delivered, but, more importantly, because it involves moral and ethical issues involving life and death on which there is no national agreement. Even a preliminary discussion on these issues has hardly begun.

Chapter 2
Rationing Medicine: Making Hard Choices Transparently

One set of illusions regarding health care in America is that we do not ration medical care and that we should not entertain doing so. The intensity of these comforting illusions is not surprising in the context of a uniquely American value system that is based on individual rights unfettered by the communitarian values that are prevalent in European countries. This emphasis on the individual is compounded by a strong belief in technological fixes and the presumption (again, largely illusory) that if only we spend enough, we can attain health and prolong life beyond its natural limits. The impact of these values is exacerbated by our tendency to look for the most painless solution to a problem and the view that somehow America can avoid the need to set strict limits common in other countries—that somehow we are different. We could not be more wrong on all points. We have finite resources and potentially infinite demands as technologies extend our capacities to intervene medically in an increasingly elderly population.

Unlike other industrialized nations that depend on explicit rationing imposed by the government, we depend on a haphazard and patently unfair mix of implicit rationing, where rationing centers on the ability to pay or to obtain insurance coverage. Any system that allows 15 percent of its population to go without health insurance is rationing. Moreover, many people with insurance experience rationing, especially of expensive medical care, through physician discretion, litigation, public relations campaigns, corporate benefits managers, and an array of other mechanisms. As stated by one wag, "We don't mind pushing people overboard; we just don't want to hear their splash."

Although we do not normally ration in the sense that national health systems do, by limiting supply or through waiting lists, our rationing is more insidious and deceptive. The question, then, is not whether we should ration medical care, but how we can best ensure a fair and equitable system of rationing—one that is more transparent and honest than what we now have. Although in an ideal world rationing would be unnecessary, because of aging populations, the proliferation of medical technologies, and heightened public expectations, rationing is essential in all health systems and can no longer be denied in the United States.

In order for such rationing to evolve, we need the contribution of both experts and the public in an open and accountable process. According to Henry Aaron, the "nation is going to have to choose between dramatically higher taxes, shredding the social safety net and … rationing," though he doubts that any of these changes will happen in the "tax-phobic" United States. Although the politics of rationing may favor continued evasion of responsibility by each of the many players, this will be more difficult to maintain in an environment where public awareness of a major crisis is mounting, as noted by Chris Ham and Angela Coulter. Because the United States is a very affluent country, until now we have been able to muddle through without a system breakdown. But the time has come where this is no longer sufficient. As aptly stated by David Seifert, "If decisions are put off until the insatiable appetite of the baby boomer generation, it will be too late to solve the cost problem."

The Need to Balance Competing Goals

Ideally, a successful health policy will provide high-quality services for all citizens on an equal basis. Moreover, it will be an efficient system with little waste and duplication and high levels of performance in all sectors. In addition to these goals of universal access, quality, and efficiency, subsidiary goals might include maximizing the patients' choices, assuring high levels of accountability, and facilitating diffusion of the newest medical technologies. Over the

> Cost containment is critical for a sustainable health system, and countries with national health or social insurance systems are much better situated to deal with the forces currently escalating health care costs. What most distinguishes the United States from other health systems is our failure to address the reality of limits that are essential in providing universal coverage at an affordable price.

last few decades, all countries have experienced a shift in balance from the goals of access and quality, predominant during the post–World War II period, to the goal of cost containment. Although access (or equity) and quality remain stated goals of most democracies, without cost containment, these other goals cannot persist. Cost containment is critical for a sustainable health system, and countries with national health or social insurance systems are much better situated to deal with the forces currently escalating health care costs. What most distinguishes the United States from other health systems is our failure to address the reality of limits that are essential in providing universal coverage at an affordable price.

To date, other Western countries have been more successful in covering all citizens at a lower per capita cost, but they have done so only by limiting the availability of high-technology medicine. As pressures emerge to expand basic care to include access to intensive curative regimes, the goal of universal coverage is threatened. The fundamental problem facing all countries, then, is how to accommodate these important but often conflicting goals. Albert Weale likens this dilemma to what logicians call an inconsistent triad: a collection of propositions, any two of which are compatible with each another but which, when viewed together in a threesome, form a contradiction. As Weale states, "Perhaps we can have only a comprehensive service of high quality, but not one available to all. Or a comprehensive service freely available to all, but not of high quality. Or a high quality service freely available to all, but not comprehensive. Each of these three possibilities defines a characteristic position in the modern debate about health care costs and organisation."

> While other countries have opted to ensure universal coverage but limit the range of health care services, the United States has opted for a system that offers high-technology, comprehensive care, but care not guaranteed to all.

While other countries have opted to ensure universal coverage but limit the range of health care services, the United States has opted for a system that offers high-technology, comprehensive care, but care not guaranteed to all. Those who have good insurance coverage have quick access to high-quality medicine with considerable freedom of choice, but at the cost of equity. In contrast, critics of national health systems argue that their comprehensive and free availability comes only at the cost of quality and subsidiary goals of choice and rapid technological diffusion. Weale suggests that though the third option—sacrificing some comprehensiveness in order to achieve at least a core range of high-quality services available to all—was a possibility when drugs were few and treatments simple, it is no longer the case because of the vast expanse of ways to spend scarce health care resources. It is not possible to meet the needs of all citizens without compromising goals. To some extent, that is what allocation and priority setting is all about: balancing to the best of our ability competing goals and demands facing the health system. In the end, what this entails is making hard choices among equally admirable goals.

In their analysis of private health spending, Drew Altman and Larry Levitt conclude that no approach the United States has used to control costs over the past four decades has had a lasting impact. Figure 2.1 shows that though the passage of Medicare and Medicaid in the mid-1960s, the institution of wage and price controls in the 1970s, the health industry's preemptive effort under threat of tough cost-containment regulations in the late 1970s, and the managed-care initiatives and threat of the Health Securities Act in the 1990s all had dramatic impact on health care costs, in every case the impact was short lived.

Neither regulation, voluntary action by the health care industry, nor managed care and market competition had a lasting impact on health care costs. Although some observers contend that the inability to control costs over time reflects a lack of resolve necessary to carry reforms through, we will not gain control over health care costs until we are ready to make tough decisions about rationing medical care.

Figure 2.1

Annual Change in Private Health Care Spending Per Capita (Adjusted for Inflation) 1961–2001

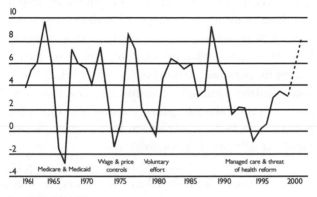

Source: Altman and Levitt, 2002.

As Altman and Levitt point out, "An equally plausible scenario is that the apparent failure of all approaches reflects the American people's uncontainable desire for the latest and best health care, and that what we will do in the future is try small things that will work at the margin, complain a lot, but ultimately pay the bill. … Indeed, history suggests that it may be folly to expect that there are any easy or magic answers to this problem."

Now is the time to confront the problem directly and make the difficult decisions needed to transform these short-term successes into a sustainable health system. The key to achieving this depends heavily on the will of the American public to rein in its thirst for medical technology and the industry's acknowledgment that unrestrained health care spending is ultimately in no one's best interests.

Allocation and Rationing

In order to accomplish the goal of maximizing health care in a sustainable way, allocation decisions are necessary at three levels. At the macro, or global, level, society must decide how much of its collective resources it is willing to devote to health care. Should we spend 8 percent of the gross domestic product, 10 percent, 15 percent, or more? What priority do we place on spending for medical care as compared to education, housing, social welfare, homeland security, and leisure, knowing that as health care gets a bigger share, other areas get a smaller one? Other concerns are the extent to which increased allocation to medical care will actually improve health of the population as opposed to the benefits of spending more in education, welfare, and housing. In other words, what are the opportunity costs of putting more into health care? Interestingly, the United States is the only Western nation that has refused to make a choice at the macro level to set limits on the proportion of its resources dedicated to health care.

> What priority do we place on spending for medical care as compared to education, housing, social welfare, homeland security, and leisure, knowing that as health care gets a bigger share, other areas get a smaller one?

Once society sets priorities at the macro level (or in the case of the United States, even if it does not choose to do so), it must decide how these resources are to be allocated among the countless competing categories of spending within health care. Again, because resources are finite, allocation here requires consideration of trade-offs. At the top of this intermediate level of allocation are decisions concerning what priority should be placed on the broad categories of health care. What takes precedence: preventive medicine, health promotion, primary care, long-term care, or individual-oriented acute medicine? Should treatment of diseases of the elderly or care of young mothers and children be given higher priority? Should higher priority be put on extending life or improving quality of life; high-incidence diseases or rare diseases; AIDS or cancer or heart disease? The decisions made here will shape, and are shaped by, what type of medicine is dominant. In the United States, the clear winners in these trade-offs have been individual-centered acute care and the elderly, whereas other countries exhibit more-balanced priorities. These trade-offs can be more or less transparent, centralized or decentralized, fair or unfair, but they will always be controversial, because they mean that some people will not get the resources they think they need.

Because we are unable to meet all the perceived health care needs of all people, ultimately rationing decisions at the individual level are unavoidable. The nature of scarcity facing all nations, driven by aging populations and the proliferation of technologies, makes it certain that the demands of individuals and groups will exceed the available resources. Collectively, it is impossible for doctors to offer all technologically feasible and clinically beneficial medicine to all patients, as they are wont to do. As noted by Leonard Fleck, there can be no health reform without health care rationing and no fair health reform without health care rationing for all.

What Is Rationing?

Some authors suggest that the term *rationing* is an archaic term used for priority setting that has given way to *resource allocation* in the last decade and will likely be called *sustainability* ten years from now as our language about this problem becomes progressively sanitized. Nevertheless, the more emotionally charged term *rationing* best reflects the emotionally charged debate on this subject. Couching the difficult decisions facing us in politically neutral terms might mollify some critics, but what is most urgently needed is a no-holds-barred debate over where we as a society should be going, and rationing health care must be central to it.

Even among those who agree that rationing is necessary, there is considerable disagreement and equivocation as to what it means. Some include macroallocation, allocation within health care, and allocation at the individual level, whereas Arnold Relman adds the dimensions of limits and deliberation in defining rationing as "the deliberate and systematic denial of certain kinds of services, even when they are known to be beneficial, because they are deemed too expensive." Meanwhile, David Hadron and Robert Brook stress the aspect of inequity. Clark Havighurst defines rationing as "the explicit denial of health care services to people who could benefit from them"; Victor Fuchs as "withholding beneficial services whether or not they are necessary"; and Alan Maynard as "a failure to offer care, or the denial of care, from which patients would benefit." All specify that rationing must entail a denial of beneficial services. Finally, Peter Ubel defines it as "any implicit or explicit mechanisms that allow people to go without beneficial services," suggesting a broad array of possible means by which rationing might be carried out.

Building from these definitions, we define rationing as the denial of a treatment to a particular patient who would benefit from it. This could be any type of treatment, but most often it is an expensive procedure or drug. Whatever specific form it takes, rationing policy always results in the situation where potentially beneficial treatment is denied to identifiable people on cost grounds. As noted by Barbara Russell, control is a central aspect of any rationing scheme. This aspect is the most contentious in America because it raises the question of control by whom. Concern is heightened when the process of rationing is done without transparency, as in the United States, where it is largely covert, implicit, and often concealed. In denial, we are forced to rely on smoke and mirrors in order to perpetuate the illusion that we, unlike other countries, do not ration. Another strategy is to blame others for constraints. Some observers contend that scarcity is a fabrication of those interests that benefit from it, and thus any subsequent limits are unwarranted and unjustified. This, we will see, is a central theme in the attacks on managed care and other cost-containment strategies. Given the huge economic stakes in health care and questionable actions of the drug companies and others, it is quite easy to sell conspiracy theories to the American public regarding attempts to ration medical resources.

Once rationing is accepted as necessary, the question becomes one of how to implement it. How do we ensure legitimacy and impartiality without compromising success? Furthermore, if resources are to be focused on the provision of *appropriate* health care, who defines this and how is it defined? And what are the criteria for rationing—total lives saved, life-years saved, or quality-of-life years saved? Because there are no clear answers and because rationing is so entangled with problems of cost containment and efficiency, its implementation is very divisive. As a result, each country's health system relies on a different combination of mechanisms. These mechanisms range from ability to pay; planned inconveniences, such as long office waiting times and complicated paperwork; gatekeeping that requires referral from a general practitioner to gain access to a specialist; a core-services package; efficiency and effectiveness controls; financial incentives and disincentives for physicians and/or patients; partial reimbursement rates; and clinical triage through waiting lists.

For our purposes, the principal distinction among rationing types is between explicit and implicit rationing. Although the definitions vary, explicit rationing usually entails decisions made by an administrative authority as to the amounts and types of resources to be made available to eligible populations and individuals, whereas implicit rationing depends on a combination of financial incentives and strategies to reduce expenditures. Although any effective system will rely on a mix of implicit and explicit approaches, rationing must be open and explicit. In contrast, some observers believe that explicit rationing is likely to be inequitable and will intensify dissatisfaction and perceived deprivation.

Another distinction that overlaps with the explicit/implicit one is supply-side versus demand-side rationing. Supply-side rationing is explicit rationing as practiced in national health systems and relies on setting strict limits from the top on medical facilities, equipment, and staffs. Moreover, general practitioners serve a gatekeeper role and deflect patients from overloading the system, while queues are used to structure the distribution of resources. In contrast, demand-side rationing, which is practiced in the United States, begins with excess hospital capacity and an oversupply of specialists and relies on informal schemes to reduce demand. However, because the system has the capacity to perform any procedure, people with adequate insurance or resources are unlikely to acquiesce to artificially imposed constraints on access. Moreover, demand-side rationing is more susceptible to personal appeals for coverage and is difficult to sustain politically. As a result of these systematic differences, there is substantially more supply-side rationing of high technologies in other countries than is politically feasible in the individualistic U.S. culture, which views supply-side constraints as socialized medicine. A related distinction is between price and non-price rationing. Price rationing, which is endemic in the United States, denies health care to people who cannot afford it or lack adequate third-party coverage. In contrast, non-price rationing, usually in combination with supply-side controls, theoretically denies certain medical resources to all people, even those who have the means to afford them.

Rationing also has been proposed as a means of guaranteeing every citizen a basic level of health care by excluding from coverage those treatments outside a defined package. This rationing by exclusion is explicit in that it identifies specific services and treatments that will not be supplied, at least to certain groups. For instance, although the Canada Health Act of 1984 guarantees health services to all citizens, it specifically excludes most adult dental services, optometry, physiotherapy, osteopathy, ambulance, dietetics, hearing aids, psychology, pharmaceuticals, and other ancillary services, except when provided in hospitals. Also, as budgets tighten, descheduling, or exclusion, of services is undertaken through negotiation with providers. Similarly, the public or private insurer can specify a set of core services or spending priorities.[1] The most detailed prioritization system was adopted in Oregon in the 1990s. Under this politically courageous plan, the state created a list of disorders ranked in descending order from those most to least economically worthwhile. By limiting the number of services normally covered under Medicaid, Oregon was able to extend access to individuals who previously were ineligible, though not without considerable public outcry and numerous lawsuits.

Rationing by exclusion has been criticized as price rationing because those with the ability to pay can obtain the services in the private market whereas those who cannot must do without. Other problems include inconsistencies in what conditions are included and diagnostic creep, which occurs when doctors manipulate diagnoses to ensure they fall within the included list. Core service or other prioritizing schemes also can lead to political pressures to add dramatic, often lifesaving interventions for specific individuals when services that have traditionally been supported are eliminated from the list.

One highly controversial issue is bedside rationing. It is controversial because it pits the traditional doctor-patient relationship against broader community interests in the distribution of collective resources. This friction clearly exemplifies the conflict between the moral levels introduced in Chapter 1. Although a doctor's first concern

---

[1]Although intuitively attractive, a major problem with a core-services approach is that there is little evidence it can be made to work (Klein, 1998). For instance, New Zealand set up the Core Services Committee in 1992 with the objective of implementing a core-services strategy to ration health services. However, after extensive public consultation and research, it concluded that a specific list of funding priorities with exclusion of specific treatment categories was politically untenable and opted instead to continue services currently funded.

is his or her patient, doctors function in society and thus have a responsibility to ensure an equitable distribution of community resources. Although in a perfect world doctors would promote their patients' best interests without regard to cost, in a world of finite resources they cannot enjoy this luxury. Peter Ubel suggests that though it is morally problematic, no acceptable rationing plan can succeed without bedside rationing. Bedside rationing is indispensable if we hope to reduce the use of extremely costly health care services that bring tiny health benefits. Furthermore, such pressures are not new. As Ubel explains, "If health care rationing was really to be avoided at all costs, we would have a nearly infinite supply of ambulances. ... Practicing medicine and making health care policy have always required tough decisions about how much health care to make available to whom and how much of society's resources should be directed to health care versus other important social goals." Whether or not a patient should be informed of bedside rationing is a subject of contention among health care experts.

For any rationing to work, there has to be enough inherent flexibility so that physicians can treat each patient appropriately. Doctors need to be more aggressive in trimming marginally beneficial health care services if there is to be any hope of controlling medical inflation, but will likely only do so through policies that mandate it.

In a 2002 survey of more than 5,000 members of the Society of Critical Care Medicine, more than two-thirds of the respondents indicated their willingness to practice bedside rationing by withholding from one patient a medication, test, or service that is in limited supply in order to give it to a patient who might benefit more. In addition, more than half of these doctors reported routinely withholding medications, tests, or services from patients when they felt that costs outweighed the potential benefit. According to Mitchell Levy, chair of Brown University's Values, Ethics, and Rationing in Critical Care, "The survey basically showed that a high percentage of physicians ration and, at the same time, feel badly that they do. You have people making decisions at the bedside on resource allocation in a relatively haphazard way, not a measured way."

Why Is Rationing So Problematic in the United States?

With all the evidence pointing toward the need for explicit rationing, what factors explain the failure of Americans to face this issue? Who is to blame? Unfortunately, there is much blame to go around, thus making the task of instituting rationing all the more difficult. Forces in opposition to rationing include politicians who overpromise; drug companies, big medicine, and a medical research community whose lifeblood is continual expansion of profit-making medical technologies; physicians who cannot say no to patients and are paid more to provide more care; tort lawyers who argue negligence when not all that is possible is done for their client; and patients and their families who demand everything that might help be done because cost should be of no concern if a third party is paying for it. Every element of U.S. health care drives it to deliver more and more. Each of these forces is mutually reinforcing, and all point back to the prevailing individualistic values of Americans. In combination, they constitute a formidable force for the status quo and a powerful obstruction in the way of genuine health care reform, in particular rationing.

As noted by Stuart Altman et al., any limitation on health spending will be met by strong resistance from groups that are negatively affected. "If the past decades have taught us anything, it is that the pressure to use medical technologies up to the point that they have no marginal value is very strong, and as a result, the long-term spending growth trend may appear to be inevitable." Although it was primarily health care providers who fought the constraints imposed on them by government in the 1970s and patients and consumer groups who were the most vocal protesters against the limitations imposed by managed-care plans in the 1990s, the response of the political system was similar in both cases. Under pressure, it caved in to the protests. In the earlier period, the federal government and most states eliminated health care price-control systems. In the 1990s, these governments imposed substantial regulatory and legal restrictions against constraints set by managed-care plans. For Altman et al., these reactions of the political system suggest that it has lacked the will to stay in the background when the negative consequences of any limits on growth become apparent. Certainly, there are always negative consequences to one group or another from reduced spending, but there are also positive consequences. However, the lessons of recent history demonstrate that the groups feeling the negative consequences win the political battle and force the government to restrict the use of those weapons that have been most effective in curtailing spending growth.

Politics

It is natural for politicians to want to please their constituents and be reelected. As such, they are beholden to those interests with political power and to the values of their constituents. In the United States, this means that politicians of both parties are likely to place high priority on protecting individual rights (including wide freedom of choice), free enterprise, and the private sector, and to favor minimal government intrusion in these areas. Moreover, with a few notable exceptions such as Governor John Kitzhaber in Oregon, they tend to overpromise and avoid talking limits. Not surprisingly then, the term *rationing* is a lightning rod for those who oppose or fear limits on medicine. Often the attack is on the word itself, with little relevance to substance. Any officials who dare set or propose to establish boundaries are attacked as instituting rationing. As a result, they avoid at all costs being seen as advocating any form of rationing and use this morally charged term only in a negative context.

Reinforcing the hesitancy to challenge entrenched interests, politicians are particularly attuned to the interests of the elderly, who have much political clout and feel most fervently about health care. The American Association of Retired Persons is a formidable political force and an outspoken opponent of rationing health services. As a result, explicit attacks such as those of Congressman Jeff Miller (R-FL) at the Health Security Act hearings are a typical response to rationing: "First of all, we have global budgets and price controls and this amounts to explicitly rationing health care. ... Seniors are the ones most victimized by rationing of health care. In other countries where they have socialized medicine, in Great Britain, for example, they ration health care. ... " In addition, there is a propensity of elected officials to favor the rights and interests of the current electorate at the expense of future generations.

Politicians are well aware that Americans are most concerned with the present, thus policies that require immediate sacrifices for future benefits are viewed as politically risky. Overall, then, there are no inherent rewards for rationing or setting limits that fail to offer immediate benefits to offset any perceived losses, and little if any concern for future generations. David Rosenbaum described this situation concisely in *The New York Times*: "So this is the conundrum for politicians. Their constituents will not accept the rationing of their medical treatment. People do not want to be told that good health has a price. On the other hand, neither the politicians nor their constituents want to pay the higher taxes or higher health insurance premiums required for unlimited health care."

According to Jeanne Scott, although many health care leaders at least privately acknowledge that American health care is almost certainly headed for such a system, rationing has long been a "third-rail issue." Poll-sensitive politicians and fainthearted academics have conspicuously avoided touching that rail, unwilling to openly suggest that the nation may require some type of rationing to preserve its health care system. Because the United States cannot continue to pay the same level of benefits to everyone who demands his or her full share of the social contract, we must either break the contract or rewrite it. Scott suggests that "In fairness to our children and grandchildren, we should rewrite it now rather than later." To do so, political leaders must take a stand, no matter how unpopular it might be initially.

Economic Forces

The over $2 trillion spent on health care gives entrenched interests, including doctors, drug companies, medical manufacturers, investors, insurance companies, and hospital corporations, a powerful incentive to maintain the status quo. It must be remembered that though out-of-control health care spending might be a crisis for society, it is an economic boon for many. This is one of the reasons economists still disagree as to whether increased spending for health care is healthy for the economy. Predictably,

> It must be remembered that though out-of-control health care spending might be a crisis for society, it is an economic boon for many.

there are many pressures from the medical research and drug industry against setting limits on diffusion of expensive, often-unproven innovations. Any efforts to rationalize this process are labeled as obstructionist, unwarranted rationing. For those who prosper by health care spending, rationing is bad news indeed.

Substantial resources are expended by the industry to extend use of its products. For example, buoyed by the 1997 federal policy change that allowed pharmaceutical companies to market their drugs directly to consumers through the mass media, they have pursued aggressive advertising blitzes and drastically expanded the demand for these costly medications beyond the original pools of patients. Moreover, direct marketing has increased pressure on physicians to overprescribe these drugs due to pressure from patients. In some cases, as evidenced by two of the most highly marketed drugs, Vioxx and Celebrex ($71 million was spent to market Celebrex for the first nine months of 2004 alone), mass marketing has led to the widespread use of these costly drugs by patients who could get the same pain benefits from over-the-counter drugs at a fraction of the cost. Not only has this wasted money, but it also has turned hype into false hope. In other cases, such as with Viagra, which Medicare approved for funding in 2005, mass marketing has also put pressure on providers to pay the costs, thus again raising costs. As noted by Tom Schatz, president of Citizens Against Government Waste, in response to Medicare coverage of impotence drugs, "Not to stiff the elderly from having a little fun, but asking Uncle Sam to pay for the romance of 76 million baby boomers will quicken the impending collapse of Medicare."

One of the clearest examples of the extent to which companies have a stake in expanding health care is the costly ($6,800 per treatment) drug Xigris, which was approved by a deeply divided FDA advisory panel in late 2001 to treat severe sepsis, which kills about 250,000 people a year. Worried about the drug's high cost and side effects, hospitals began writing narrow guidelines for its use, leading some doctors to question whether patients were being subjected to hospital rationing policies, and at times dying. With Xigris sales far below expectations, its producer, Eli Lilly, fueled the debate by awarding a $1.8 million grant for a study of rationing practices, successfully lobbying for a special reimbursement of half the drug's cost by Medicare, hiring public-relations firms to shape a rationing debate strategy, and rallying sympathetic patients and doctors. Lilly's case was strengthened by a survey of intensive-care doctors who found that Xigris was the most widely rationed drug: 27 percent said they had been forced to withhold Xigris, and 43 percent said they likely could be. Adding to the controversy was the fact that the survey was conducted by a doctor who consults with Lilly. Moreover, some experts say the drug is not widely used because doctors simply aren't convinced it works. In a clinical trial of 1,690 patients, 25 percent of Xigris patients died, compared with 31 percent of those on standard treatment, which typically cost less than $50 a day. After a group of scientists published a critical assessment of Xigris, Lilly rebutted the criticisms as without merit and stated that the denial of the drug to desperately ill patients is unethical.

The Medical Profession

The medical profession is far from monolithic when it comes to rationing, though most clinicians find themselves uncomfortable being required to set priorities or affected by the decisions of others about priorities. G. Caleb Alexander et al., for instance, found that many physicians faced with scarcity on a daily basis are reluctant to acknowledge the ways that limited health care resources influence their decisions. They believe that such decisions should be left to policy makers, who are removed from patient care. Although it is not surprising that physicians frequently deny that health care scarcity influences their practice, this counters the reality that their decisions often require trade-offs of limited resources. This denial of scarcity serves as a barrier to containing costs and developing fair allocation systems because those making the ultimate decision misperceive the need to set limits. It may also contribute to the willingness of physicians to lie to obtain marginal benefits for their patients in practices such as diagnostic creep. Physicians have found ways to "game" the system in response to cost-containment efforts of managed-care organizations with substantial public support of this practice. Thus the actual need to contain health care costs may be denied by attributing cost-containment pressures to greedy managed-care organizations. But accountability for rationing choices also requires careful governance of the agents of medical care—doctors—who judge the health needs of competing patients. Without the support of the medical profession, any attempt at explicit rationing is doomed to failure.

The Legal System

Given its emphasis on individual rights, it is no surprise that the United States has the world's most extensive medical liability system. Although the medical community claims medical malpractice suits represent a crisis needing reform, trial lawyers and consumer groups argue that the real problem is the failure of the medical profession to discipline bad doctors and that any attempt to limit awards will undermine the rights of individuals to redress wrongs in a court of law. Although the direct cost of malpractice insurance is considerable, its indirect impact is even more profound. In addition to the added cost of maintaining legal council in medical facilities, virtually every medical decision is made within a legal milieu and under threat of litigation. This in turn leads to defensive medicine, where doctors order diagnostic tests and therapeutic measures that are of marginal or no benefit simply to avoid potential litigation. Although there is considerable debate over the full costs of defensive medicine, it adds significantly to health spending. Any attempts to ration medical services—for example, the refusal of insurance companies to cover organ transplants and other expensive interventions—are met with threats of legal action. Although many of these attempts have failed, in some cases courts have ordered coverage, with a sobering effect on cost containment.

With regard to Health Maintenance Organizations (HMOs), this environment might be changing in light of a 9–0 vote in the Supreme Court that recognized inherent limits of health care provision and the inevitability of rationing. In *Pegram v. Herdrich*, the Court reversed a lower court's finding involving a patient's right to sue her HMO for limiting treatment due to cost concerns. According to the Court, employees who accept the health insurance offered have no guarantee they will receive all the care unlimited money could provide. The Court was not willing to upset this cost-containment system by allowing "wholesale attacks" on HMOs. In the words of Justice David Souter, writing for the Court:

> No HMO organization could survive without some incentive connecting physician reward with treatment rationing. The essence of an HMO is that salaries and profits are limited by the HMO's fixed membership fees. ... Since inducement to ration care goes to the very point of any HMO scheme, and rationing necessarily raises some risks while reducing others ... any legal principle purporting to draw a line between good and bad HMOs would embody, in effect, a judgment about socially acceptable medical risk. ... But such complicated fact finding and such a debatable social judgment are not wisely required of courts unless for some reason resort cannot be had to the legislative process, with its preferable forum for comprehensive investigations and judgments of social value, such as optimum treatment levels and health care expenditure.

The Public and Its Advocates

Despite protestations from the Clinton administration that the Health Security Act would not entail rationing, opponents playing on the public's fear of rationing were able to soundly defeat it by linking it to rationing. The public responded true to form—with strong rejection. There is always a concern on the part of the public about getting the care they need and the belief that rationing does not occur—and if it does, it is wrong. Any attempts to set limits are immediately met by condemnation of rationing. Schering-Plough CEO Fred Hassan played on this concern at a meeting of the American Heart Association when he complained that certain government programs and aspects of managed care were constraining the role of physicians to do what is best for their patients. Hassan stated that these "restrictions and constraints are driven by a short-term goal of saving costs by rationing health care." Likewise, the Association of American Physicians and Surgeons established an initiative to create an awareness of alternatives to the "unconscionable government rationing of care to seniors":

> Up until now, government bureaucrats have said they'll decide how to ration care—that seniors are too stupid or feeble to decide with their doctors what medical care is best for them. This is an important and overdue acknowledgement that the government has no right to say you can't spend your own money even if it means saving your own life.

Interestingly, they failed to mention that the rationing they were referring to was of the government's money, not the patient's.

Others brand any policy that cuts health care funding as rationing. In a *Jackson (TN) Sun* editorial titled "Coming Soon to an Insurance Plan Near You: Health

Care Rationing," Tom Bohs finds it "inconceivable" that a liberal Democratic governor had the audacity to set rules that limit hospital stays, doctor visits, and drug prescriptions funded by the TennCare program, which has blown out the Tennessee budget in recent years.

> Health care rationing has come to Tennessee. ... Health care rationing means this: You get so much health care service, then it stops. When you have exhausted your allocated ration of health care services, you're on your own. Need another day in the hospital? Forget it. Need one more trip to the doc to make certain the cure he gave you is working? You and the doc are on your own. Need another prescription to make that health-enhancing pharmaceutical cocktail work? Nope.

Similar apprehension is reflected in the concern of a letter writer to the *St. Louis Post-Dispatch*: "Despite exorbitant health insurance premiums, I and others have our health care rationed daily. My HMO tells me what doctors I may see, what hospitals I may use, what drugs I may take. ... I call this rationing. One doctor said to my husband, 'Let's start with the cheapest test.' Not the appropriate or needed test, but the cheapest. ... Isn't this rationing?"

Often, rationing is presented as a direct assault on individual rights. Emily Duncan, for example, contends that society has an obligation to provide the basics, including decent health care, for all people, without rationing. "Health care is a human right. Regardless of whether an individual can pay for it or not, they are entitled to it. Health care should be free." Presumably, then, all citizens have an unfettered right to all the health care they need. Although this statement appears extreme, a survey by the Opinion Research Corporation of 1,020 adults in 2004 found that 67 percent of the respondents thought that health care coverage should be a "guarantee," with 78 percent agreeing that health care is a necessity like water and power that requires government regulation to ensure benefits. The study's authors concluded that Americans are ready for reform, but the data demonstrate little support for rationing. Instead, the notion of limits is firmly rejected: 71 percent disagreed with the idea that patients who have HMO coverage should have fewer rights to care, and 83 percent thought patients denied coverage for "medically necessary" treatment should have the right to sue for damages. Furthermore, Claudia Schur et al. found that those people reporting the worst health status are most likely to reject cost-containment strategies that might interfere in their ability to obtain health care services. Although they are least receptive to restrictive managed-care tactics, they are also the least willing to pay a higher deductible or premium to avoid them. As reflected in these polls, it is clear that for the American public, the crisis in health care can be resolved only by less-expensive health care coverage, not less-expensive health care. Similarly, other opinion surveys show that though at least 40 percent of respondents cite health care as the most important problem facing the government, even larger percentages favor increased spending on medical technology.

American patients also have come to expect a different standard of care. In contrast to many other countries where physicians spend little time with patients, such

> Claudia Schur et al. found that those people reporting the worst health status are most likely to reject cost-containment strategies that might interfere in their ability to obtain health care services.

conduct would be unacceptable here. Moreover, one is struck by the comparatively Spartan conditions in hospitals in other nations. In the United States, amenities commonly include satellite TV, DVD libraries, bedside phones, wide menu choices, and tastefully decorated rooms. These extras have little appreciable impact on health but add substantially to the costs. One hospital in Sarasota, Florida, for instance, recently added an "enhanced amenity wing" where "you will experience a hospital stay like no other." Amenities include a full-time concierge service; a "design-enhanced" private suite with custom convertible sleeper for guests, a refrigerator/ freezer, a personal computer with Internet access, and an armoire; a private dining room with hardwood floors and a "chef-enhanced menu" for patient and guests; a gourmet "Java Joint"; a private elevator; and daily fresh flowers, newspapers, and healing-touch therapy.

Public opposition to rationing is also unmistakable in its response to HMOs. HMOs were established to constrain costs by setting limits to care so that more-explicit rationing could be forestalled. For the first several years, they did this, and the rise in health costs slowed. But, as *The New York Times*'s David Rosenbaum notes, "The public began to complain about all the rules limiting the services they could receive—about the rationing." Movies and television shows took up the theme of HMOs as the enemy of the people, and eventually these complaints led to a proposed patients' bill of rights aimed at overruling the very factors that made HMOs effective. As a result of employee displeasure at the restrictions, employers gradually made the plans less restrictive. Similarly, hospitals and physicians fought the limits and went through a wave of mergers to give themselves more power. Not surprisingly, as a result of weakening managed care, insurance premiums rose 10.9 percent in 2001, 12.9 percent in 2002, and 13.9 percent in 2003. Once again, the citizenry opted for more-immediate access to a full range of specialists of their choice and to the latest medical technologies, roundly rejecting the notion of limits—of the dreaded rationing. John Pulskamp et al. illustrate this bitterness when they state: "The HMOs have proved to be too greedy, extracting billions in the form of windfall profits by withholding [rationing] appropriate medical care to millions of customers" and have been "instrumental in the transformation of doctors into puppets of the insurers."

At its base, the moral debate about rationing pits individual choice against communal interests. In the United States, as opposed to other Western nations, the individual always trumps the community. Although all countries are rooted in a system where the healthy are expected to help pay for the sick, according to Humphrey Taylor, chairman of the Harris Poll, in America "that social contract is fraying." Americans expect to take as much out of a health plan as they put in and are not concerned with creating a pool of money to pay for the small number of very sick patients. Likewise, Allan Buchanan contends that the cries of unjust treatment by members of managed-care plans who faced rationing illustrates the absence of a shared conception of justice for determining to what health care resources a person has a just claim. He argues that if they are unhappy with this state of affairs, they must engage in public deliberations that can create and legitimate a shared conception of health care justice. For such legitimization to occur, however, the safe and indifferent middle class in managed-care plans will have to address the problem of the uninsured.

Interestingly, many of the proponents of a single-payer system are the strongest opponents of rationing; in fact, they argue that only moves to such a system will allow us to escape rationing. This is unrealistic because universal coverage is workable only when restraints on breadth of coverage are imposed. Single-payer countries are more successful in providing universal coverage with lower per capita costs than the United States only because they constrain the availability of high-technology medicine. Once they broaden basic care to include unlimited access to intensive curative regimes, they lose this advantage. The reality is that no nation can afford to do everything for everybody. Therefore, national health systems rely heavily on setting supply-side controls through global budgets and national fee structures whereas social insurance systems use contractual arrangements to limit what individuals get. Because these countries have more communitarian- and solidarity-based value systems (probably explaining why they have universal coverage in the first place), their populations are much more willing to live (or die) with what Americans would see as an unfair system, in other words, one that rations medicine.

As noted by Daniel Callahan, acceptance of the idea of rationing is a necessary first step toward universal health insurance: "Commentators have argued that reform of the health care system should come before any effort to ration. On the contrary, rationing and reform cannot be separated. The former is the key to the latter, just as rationing is the key to universal health insurance." Every single-payer health system has at its core some form of health care rationing, including strict limits on expensive care, such as organ transplants, chemotherapy, and bone marrow transplants, and long waiting times for elective surgeries, such as joint replacements. This is not to say that rationing is not a highly divisive issue in all countries, as evidenced by the huge number of articles written on rationing in the United Kingdom alone. The point is that it is an issue open to discourse in other countries. In the United States, on the other hand, rationing is rejected out of hand as something to be avoided at all costs, an unethical imposition of limits on something that should have none. Clearly, our one-dimensional view of medical ethics with its focus on the needs of the individual patient at the exclusion of broader duties blinds us to the

> In the United States ... rationing is rejected out of hand as something to be avoided at all costs, an unethical imposition of limits on something that should have none.

realities of scarcity. It is ironic that though large majorities of Americans favor guaranteed coverage such as that offered by National Health Service (NHS) systems, very few are willing to even listen to arguments for the rationing that must accompany such reform.

Strategies Short of Explicit Rationing Will Not Resolve the Long-Term Health Crisis

Some pundits contend that this "crisis" is a myth and that we would have sufficient funds to resolve health care funding problems if we just allocated more societal resources to health care. They claim that a reordering of spending priorities and the designation of special status to health care would provide adequate funds to handle the problems of health care allocation. Regrettably, these arguments are contradicted by two factors. First, there is little evidence of a large cache of funding that can be transferred to health care. Already, health care siphons off resources from other social programs and is the biggest growth area in most state budgets. Second, history indicates that the appropriation of additional funds to medicine often exacerbates rather than resolves the problems. Because health care needs and demands are virtually unlimited and funding sources are not, shifting higher proportions of the GDP or the federal budget to medical ends simply serves to postpone that inevitable point at which constraints must be imposed.

Cutting Waste and Inefficiency

Another line of argument that represents a last gasp against the need for explicit rationing suggests that the costs of health care can be effectively contained by making efficiency improvements through managed competition, reduction of administrative costs, and elimination of unnecessary and wasteful care. Surveys have found that a majority of the American public believes that the problems we face are caused by the waste, inefficiency, and greed of insurance companies, hospitals, physicians, pharmaceutical companies, and malpractice lawyers, all problems that can be resolved without making personal sacrifices. Because of this myopia, the public is not amenable to proposals that limit their use of medical technologies and ready access to highly trained medical specialists of their choice, or otherwise constrain their rights to health care.

Although it has been estimated that at least one-third of our health care costs might be safely relinquished by cutting waste, Henry Aaron cautions that no one really knows what the savings might be or if "practicable, politically sustainable institutional arrangements for eliminating this care can be devised." Despite this uncertainty, this approach is attractive because cutting "waste" as opposed to rationing does not signify the denial of necessary care. Medical ethicist Robert Veatch, however, rightly cautions that rationing of health care is an inevitable correlate of living in a world of finite resources and that "cutting the fat out of the system" will not be sufficient. Instead, a "true social ethic of resource allocation" is necessary. Although all efforts should be made to eliminate waste and inefficiency, there is overwhelming evidence that such steps alone will not be sufficient to avoid setting limits on our appetite for and dependence on sophisticated medical interventions.

Moreover, a major difficulty is defining what is wasteful and what is not. Waste to one person might be considered indispensable to another. For instance, a recent study reported a "disturbing rise" in the number of cancer patients receiving chemotherapy and other aggressive but futile treatment in the last days of their lives. Despite giving false hope through often painful and costly ordeals, critics argued that patients (and their families) do not like to give up, and thus the treatment should not be viewed as futile. So though we may all agree that much medical care is of doubtful benefit and that the health system has enormous waste and inefficiency, it is not possible to eliminate targeted care without controversy. Patients and their doctors are unlikely to acquiesce to the elimination of procedures that might help them on grounds they are wasteful. As noted by Theodore Marmor and David Boyum:

However untested, therapies will always be sought by
patients wanting to improve their lives, while doctors
themselves will want to employ them. Monetary incentives certainly play a role, but physicians are also guided
by a special professional ethic. ... there is little likelihood
that either of the intimate partners in the doctor-patient
relationship will ever perceive a significant proportion of
medical treatments as "wasteful."

In addition, given the near limitless expandability
of the medical industry and the large monetary stakes
involved, it is questionable whether such savings could
forestall difficult allocation decisions for more than a
short time. Although some savings will occur if outcome
studies result in the elimination of wasteful practices and
the system is made more efficient, the dominant underlying force responsible for rising medical expenditures—
technological advances—will persist. William Schwartz
and Daniel Mendelson estimate that efficiency gains are
not likely to reduce the rise in costs by more than 1.5
percent annually, and they conclude that much more
stringent measures are necessary to make substantial
reductions: "Some portion of the increase in costs due
to technology may be restrained by devices and drugs
that can accomplish a given task at a lower cost. But
unless fiscal constraints are severe enough to discourage
innovation, the flood of new technologies is likely to
overwhelm any savings resulting from a new concern for
cost-effectiveness over the next decade."

Henry Aaron agrees that moves to cut waste and inefficiency will not materially slow the growth of overall
health care spending. First, even if inappropriate therapies
are eliminated, the symptoms that occasioned therapy in

the first place call for some other form of treatment. Second, effectiveness research itself is costly, complex, and time consuming, and although clear-cut results might emerge, many outcomes studies reveal mixed results in which a therapy is superior in some respects and inferior in others. Counteracting these efforts, large numbers of new medical devices, procedures, and drugs will come into use, most of which will tend to drive up overall costs, and major new initiatives such as stem-cell research and biotechnology will drastically add to the costs. Therefore, any measures short of rationing beneficial services and slowing technological diffusion are unlikely to resolve the problem of rising costs.

A related proposed means of avoiding rationing is by eliminating the inefficiency of our fragmented payer system and the administrative costs it places on hospitals. There is no doubt that the administrative cost of our health insurance system is indefensibly high. For every dollar the insurance industry pays in claims, almost 18 cents is spent on marketing, administration, and other overhead expenses. In addition to these direct costs of administration, the estimated hospital costs driven by the need to meet reporting requirements of managed-care organizations and insurance carriers range from $41 billion to $47 billion per year. Schwartz and Mendelson note, however, that dramatic reductions are difficult to achieve because administrative costs already have been reduced over the last decade. They estimate that hospital administrative costs could realistically save approximately $5 billion annually, a large amount, but certainly not enough to make a dent in mushrooming health care costs. Although lowering administrative costs should receive high priority, promises of huge savings must be met with skepticism.

Dependence on the Marketplace

Similarly, many economists place considerable faith in market forces to constrain health care costs through competition. The fallacy of this approach is that the health care market contains none of the self-selecting mechanisms that normally work to check market excesses. In order for an efficient, market-based health care system to work, several conditions are essential: (1) all decisions must be made by the consumer, (2) the consumer must know the value and costs of the goods he or she is contemplating purchasing, and (3) the consumer must pay the full cost and receive the full value of the goods she or he chooses to buy. Not one of these conditions is present in the market for health care services. First, no medical decisions are solely that of the patient: ultimately the patient's choice is heavily conditioned and constrained by the providers. Second, most patients are unable to judge the value of the care they get. As a result, health care providers have enormous discretion in deciding both the type and cost of care provided. Moreover, the emotional and often urgent nature of medical decisions undercuts the patient's ability to be a rational shopper. Also, it does not follow that more-informed consumers of health care will buy at a lower cost. In fact, evidence suggests that knowledge often leads to higher costs because informed patients tend to be more demanding.

The major reason that patients are unlikely to be prudent consumers, however, is that third-party payment, whether public or private, means that the potential consumer pays only a fraction of the costs, if any. Third-party payment is accompanied by overconsumption, as neither the patient nor the physician has an incentive to economize when a third party is paying the bill. The term *moral hazard* is used to refer to the behavioral changes that occur when people are put in a position to

Third-party payment is accompanied by overconsumption, since neither the patient nor the physician has an incentive to economize when a third party is paying the bill.

spend or risk the funds of others. The bottom line is that unless there are strong disincentives, people will want more when someone else is paying for the service. Mary Ann Baily describes moral hazard as follows:

> Insurance provides subscribers with valuable peace of mind; however, it introduces inefficiency into decisions about the use of care. When insurance pays the bill, people consume health care as if it were free, rather than weighing the benefit of a particular service against its cost (as they do for the other goods and services they buy and consume). The health care is not free, of course, since the premium must be set high enough to cover the total cost of the health care provided to the entire group.

Although the moral hazard problem is by no means unique to health care, it is a major consideration in the development of fair rationing strategies.

Consumer-Directed Health Plans

A fashionable demand-based strategy for reducing health care costs without having to resort to rationing is to give patients an incentive to use less or to provide tiered premium strategies that let the consumers pick their own package of benefits. The former version is based on the notion that health care services are overutilized, in part because of the moral hazard, and that with the proper financial incentives, individuals will opt for less. Driving this movement is the view that individuals can best make their own choices among health care through vehicles such as health savings accounts (HSAs), and that when allowed to do so, they will opt to use less, thus saving the system money. Other monikers for this approach are *medical savings accounts, health reimbursement arrangements*, and *consumer-directed strategies*.

Consumer-driven strategies, often presented as empowering health care consumers, take many forms but typically include a high-deductible policy that is offered with either a health reimbursement account or a health savings account. This is the approach of the Bush administration plan, where consumers who purchase a catastrophic insurance policy can set aside a tax-free amount equal to their deductible in a portable HSA with unused balances rolled over from year to year. Supporters say this plan will give workers and their families an incentive to be more frugal users of health care and that the lower premiums on high-deductible plans will make coverage affordable for the uninsured and small businesses. Critics counter it is nothing but an attempt to shift the risks, costs, and problems from employers to individuals.

Although there is considerable evidence that such approaches reduce usage, critics argue that such savings are short-run at best because they encourage people to forego needed care, thus increasing costs later. Moreover, critics suggest that though such plans will be most attractive to young, healthy workers, older and sicker people will be left out. The key empirical study on cost sharing, the RAND Health Insurance Experiment, randomly assigned individuals to insurance plans ranging from free care for all services to those with widely varying copayments. In the cost-sharing plans, everyone was given a lump sum payment of maximum out-of-pocket costs ($1,000) less the maximum out-of-pocket under their current coverage, which they could spend as they chose. Unsurprisingly, this study confirmed that consumers use fewer services when they share the costs. Moreover, though initial findings suggested no negative impact on health status, later studies found that cost sharing reduced the likelihood of receiving effective care because people did not want to spend their own money and did not get timely treatment. For instance, a recent Commonwealth Fund report raises major concerns about relying on such strategies to address the long-term problems facing U.S. health care, because they might simply defer the health costs.

Savings by Reducing Costs at End of Life

America expends more medical resources on terminally ill patients and intervenes more aggressively at the end of life than other nations. Thus, dying in the United States is expensive: on average, 18 percent of one's lifetime health care costs are spent during the last year of life, three to eight times that of other years. Of this amount, 77 percent is spent in the last six months and almost one-third in the last thirty days. Moreover, 29 percent of Medicare and Medicaid payments are made on behalf of the 5 percent of beneficiaries who die in a given year. And, of all the patients who enter ICUs, a significant number die either during their stay or shortly after discharge, often at great expense. Based on statistics of this sort, some observers suggest that we can save huge amounts of health dollars if only we limit care for terminally ill patients. The argument is that by eliminating intensive (and expensive) treatment for terminal patients, resources could be released for patients who will live, thus allowing us to avoid explicit rationing of beneficial or needed treatments.

One salient movement over the last several decades has been the encouragement of advance directives (ADs) in the form of living wills or durable powers of attorney. Although ADs were established ostensibly to empower patients to take control over medical decision-making and ensure their autonomy, the resource allocation dimension is readily apparent. By definition, ADs are a means of voluntarily rejecting available medical interventions, specifically regimes of aggressive treatment for terminal patients. One problem is that terminal illness is an imprecise and ambiguous term, meaning that in some cases the uncertainty of prognosis makes it impossible to predict which patients will live and which will die with the same treatment. As a result, a conservative approach to ADs will keep some patients alive beyond the desired time whereas a liberal interpretation will end treatment for some patients whose lives could have been saved.

With regard to advance directives, findings are mixed, but in general there is little evidence they produce significant aggregate cost savings. This is not surprising, because, contrary to what many believe, only a relatively small amount of costly, high-technology medicine is expended on unquestionably terminal patients: most is spent on critically ill patients. Terminally ill patients are those who have a high probability of dying in the short run, no matter what is done. In contrast, though a critically ill patient may die even with aggressive treatment, death is possible but not probable. What this means is if we really want to save significant medical resources, such

constraints must be extended to critically ill patients—
often frail, debilitated, and elderly, but not in imminent
danger of dying—who cumulatively account for far more
resources. The question, then, is how far we extend non-
treatment into the critically ill category.

This leads to the consideration of when it is acceptable to curtail futile treatment and, more fundamentally,
what constitutes a futile treatment. Like terminal illness, futility is an elusive concept, because it is difficult
to predict with certainty that a treatment will be of no
benefit to a particular patient. Some believe that on
grounds of futility, even the universal application of
CPR is indefensible, because for most patients, CPR is
a desperate measure with slender prospects of success.
Others, however, reject the concept of futility itself and
argue that it has no place in medical decision making.
The debate over futile treatment reveals two conflicting
motivations. The first is that curtailing futile treatment
protects patient autonomy and the integrity of the physicians as moral and professional agents. To force truly
futile treatment on a patient is dehumanizing. A second
motivation, however, is to save resources, as an inherent
aspect of futility is that the benefit of such treatment is
not worth the investment because it is bound to fail. The
notion of futility as wasteful thus can be used to sanction
restrictions on the allocation of resources under the guise
of patient autonomy. Under this scenario, patients could
not demand futile therapy, and society and the medical
community would be under no obligation to provide it
to those who do.

The evidence across these areas suggests that the idea
that we can avoid explicit rationing by eliminating waste,
instituting consumer-directed health plans, encouraging

advance directives, or terminating futile treatment for clearly terminal patients is largely an illusion. Although needed savings will accrue from such changes, and these changes might be inherently admirable in terms of patient empowerment and other goals, it is unlikely that they alone will be sufficient to make significant inroads into continually escalating health care costs. In order to approach savings of the magnitude needed, such care would have to be withheld from a substantially broadened population of critically ill patients. Ann Scitovsky is correct when she states: "Chronically ill patients present us with the dilemma not so much to forgo 'heroics,' but rather of when to halt ordinary care (such as treatment with antibiotics in case of infection) and sustenance." In what way, however, is this not explicit rationing? Ironically, then, though these approaches are often proffered as means of avoiding explicit rationing, they incorporate a form of surreptitious rationing by hiding it beneath the veneer of empowerment.

———

Given the combined force of opponents lined up against rationing in the face of reality, where do we go from here? How do we convince all of the potential stakeholders and users that denial of rationing is an illusion and will become more so in the coming decades? Despite the hostility toward rationing in the United States, the rationing of medical technologies is endemic. However, the customary approach to rationing practiced by health care providers, often on a price basis but not explicitly acknowledged, gives us the false impression that we do not have to make these choices. This deception, in turn, has fueled anger, directed at the bearers of the bad news, that explicit rationing is unavoidable as the baby boom generation ages. Explicit rationing of medical resources is alien to a rights-oriented value system, but ultimately there is no escape from it.

In the absence of coordinated, consistent national criteria, rationing decisions will continue to be made on an ad hoc, reactive basis through a combination of public and private mechanisms. The question, then, is not whether rationing ought to be done, but rather how we can best establish institutionalized procedures that are fair and reasonable. To this end, a first order of business is to pursue a public dialogue over societal goals and priorities that considers the preferred agents for rationing medical resources. Although reaching a consensus on the actual distribution of medical resources is likely unattainable, the goal should be to reach agreement regarding the procedures of rationing. If we can come to an agreement that the decisional criteria are fair and understand that all are bound by them, specific decisions, however difficult, might be accepted as unfortunate, but not unfair.

One of the reasons Americans reject the notion of explicit rationing is that there is no guarantee that the resources averted from them or their loved ones will be used fairly or even more efficiently elsewhere. Make a sacrifice, and someone less deserving might get *your* resources. Strict rationing by governmental mandate during World War II enjoyed strong public support because losses were compensated by the promise of freedom and security. In effect, one group of tangible benefits was replaced by valuable intangible benefits, including that of doing something important for your nation. Furthermore, this rationing affected virtually everyone, and this mutuality and inclusiveness strengthened public support. In sharp contrast, health care rationing has never enjoyed public support, in part because we depend on a marketplace that privileges the individual and pits one person against another for access to resources. As discussed earlier, our value system ensures that the collective good is secondary to the individual. We need strong leaders who can instill a sense of purpose and the importance of community found in the war experience.

Although the medical profession, the medical industry, and policy makers, among others, are important factors in moving toward a transparent rationing system, the biggest obstacle to cost-effective resource allocation today is the attitude of consumers. Although the American abhorrence at putting a price on life helps explain our stiff resistance to rationing, consumer acceptance is possible if particular checks and balances are incorporated. Our major task, then, is to convince the public that there will be a consistency and justice in the way we ration and to nurture a sense of community that transcends a "me-first" mind-set. It would be foolish to presume that moderation of expectations and demands of a public that has come to expect unlimited access to technological progress in medicine is an easy task, because at present there seems to be little political will or general inclination to constrain health care spending.

Honesty is better than silence regarding the realities of rationing. Acting as if such limitations do not exist is self-deceptive, and inevitably produces the wrong conclusions and decisions. As cogently stated by Barbara

Russell, "When confronted with 'bad news,' the ethical challenge should not center on whether to divulge or not, but rather on how to divulge. Candidly and openly facing these inescapable 'tragic choices' does require strong moral character and a supportive environment for debate, both of which can be absent within the high-stakes, adversarial setting of contemporary American politics." The unpopularity of the message should not be allowed to deter us from the task at hand, nor does it reduce the need and urgency of facing it.

Chapter 3

Individual Behavior and Age as Considerations in Rationing

In order to ensure that health care has sufficient resources
in the future, we need to begin a discourse on a variety
of dramatic cost-limiting concepts. Many solutions to
our health care crisis will likely lie far beyond our current dialogue. Not only are we as a society not currently
talking about them, they may lie beyond our imagina-
tion. The transition from the current state of health care,
which is growing at over twice the rate of inflation, to a
growth rate at or below the rate of inflation will require
concepts and actions that are now considered unacceptable. Two of the most essential but contentious areas deal
with the extent to which age and individual behavior
ought to be considerations in rationing. The data below
clearly demonstrate that the elderly and those individuals
who engage in unhealthy behavior consistently consume
a disproportionate share of the resources. Therefore, if
we are to control health care spending, we must constrain the amount of resources going to the elderly and
to people who engage in risky behavior, simply because
they consume at such high rates. We must reinstitute the
notion of individual responsibility for health, which has
given way to the right to health care, and admit we can
no longer afford to do everything that might be done
technologically for elderly people. Even though both of

these proposals are regarded as politically incorrect by critics, they are unavoidable, and ultimately fairer than the current state of affairs.

The Concentration of Health Care Costs

Rationing is complicated by the fact that the distribution of health care resources is skewed toward a small percentage of the population that accounts for a large proportion of expenditures. Accompanying the shift toward sophisticated curative care over the second half of the twentieth century, health care spending has become concentrated in a relatively small number of patients in acute-care settings. Table 3.1 demonstrates the extent of this intensifying concentration of health resources. In 1996, the top 1 percent of users in the United States accounted for 27 percent of all health care expenditures; the top 5 percent used 55 percent; and the top 10 percent used 69 percent. In contrast, only 3 percent of payments

> The majority of Americans are responsible collectively for a very small proportion of health care spending.

went to those patients in the bottom half of the population. Those in the bottom 50 percent incurred an average annual expenditure of $122 in medical costs in 1996 compared with an average expenditure of $56,459 for those in the top 1 percent. Thus, the majority of Americans are responsible collectively for a very small proportion of health care spending. Moreover, as Marc Berk and Alan Monheit note, there has been a "remarkable stability in this concentration pattern over the last three decades."

It is possible, of course, that these figures reflect the fact that though a few people become seriously ill each year and use significant resources, they are replaced by others in following years. David Mechanic, for instance,

Table 3.1

Distribution of Health Expenditures for the U.S. Population by Magnitude of Expenditures for Selected Years 1963–1996

Percent of U.S. Population Ranked by Expenditures	1963	1970	1977	1980	1987	1996
Top 1%	17%	26%	27%	29%	28%	27%
Top 2%	—	35%	38%	39%	39%	38%
Top 5%	43%	50%	55%	55%	56%	55%
Top 10%	59%	66%	70%	70%	70%	69%
Top 30%	—	88%	90%	90%	90%	90%
Bottom 50%	5%	4%	3%	4%	3%	3%

Source: Adapted from Berk and Monheit, 2001.

argues that this pattern should not be surprising, because each year only a small proportion of the population suffers critical illness, but they are not necessarily the same people who are using expensive resources in other years. Although this argument has merit, a sixteen-year longitudinal study found that approximately half of the population has few health care needs other than routine measures over their lifetime, 45 percent incur substantial health care costs at some point, and 5 percent experience extraordinary health needs and expenses throughout their lives. Anecdotal evidence from emergency rooms also reveals that a small number of repeat patients consume substantial resources over a longer term.

In a more systematic analysis of high users, Monheit found that a sizable majority of high users exhibit persistently high expenditures from one year to the next. Among the top 5 percent of spenders in 1996, for instance, approximately 30 percent remain in this percentile in 1997, and

45 percent remain in the top decile. In contrast, people with relatively low expenditures in a given year largely remain in low-expenditure percentiles. Although this high-expenditure persistence by a sizable minority of high spenders does regress to the mean over several years, people over the age of sixty-five are more likely to remain in the top decile of spenders across years. Moreover, 12.6 percent of persons in the top 1 percent of spenders and 7 percent in the top 5 percent died in 1996. Monheit also found that the expenditures by such people are disproportionately high relative to their representation in the population: the average cost of $31,828 for those who died in the top 10 percent of spenders is more than twice the overall average, whereas the $25,559 average for people who died in the top half of all spenders was six times the average for that group. No matter how the data are spread, there is considerable evidence that high users of health care constitute a minority of the population and that there is persistence in the makeup of this population, at least across the short run of several years.

If we are to gain control of health care spending, it is imperative that we know who the high users are, because little can be saved on those who use minimal or no resources each year. By and large, high users are more likely to be people with chronic medical problems who are repeatedly admitted to the hospital than people with a single cost-intensive stay. According to Monheit, people who remained in the top decile of spending over these two years "differed markedly" from those who remained in the bottom half in that they are older and "far more likely to be female." This reconfirms the fact, discovered in Berk and Monheit's study, that of those with high expenditures in 1996, 46.3 percent are elderly who as a group comprise 12.7 percent of the population. In addition to the elderly, high users of health care predominantly are identified as consistently ill individuals, many of whom have unhealthy lifestyles. Ten key risk factors, including alcohol and drug abuse, heavy smoking, obesity, sedentary lifestyles, and unhealthy diets, are particularly prominent among high users of medical care. In addition to having more frequent episodes of ill health, patients with these behaviors require more repeated hospitalizations for each episode, thus increasing the "limit cost" of the illness. This small proportion of patients, then, exerts disproportionate leverage on medical resources by repeated use of hospital facilities (see Box 3.1).

Data on the major causes of mortality reflect a shift from infectious diseases to degenerative chronic diseases linked to individual behavior (see Table 3.2). It is estimated by the Public Health Service that 50 percent of all premature deaths are associated with choices individuals make. As illustrated in Table 3.3, two factors, smoking and obesity, accounted for 35 percent of the 2.4 million deaths in 2000. Moreover, it has been estimated that 50 to 90 percent of all cancers are promoted or caused by various personal and environmental factors. Louis Sullivan notes that "Better control of fewer than ten risk factors ... could prevent between 40 and 70 percent of all premature deaths, a third of all cases of acute disability, and two-thirds of all cases of chronic disability." Although there are no accurate estimates of the health costs of premature mortality or preventable morbidity caused by imprudent behavior, it runs into the hundreds of billions of dollars annually. For instance, the National Institutes of Health estimated the costs to society of alcohol-related problems in 1992 at $148 billion. Likewise, the impact of obesity on health care spending is substantial and growing rapidly. In addition to heightened levels of diabetes, hypertension, and other health conditions among obese patients, hip and knee replacements among this group are predicted to grow by 600 percent in the coming decade. It is unlikely, given the trends in disease and illness and the massive health costs associated with certain individual behaviors, that we can make major inroads on the health financing crisis without altering behavior of individuals.

These data have important implications for the financing of health services on several grounds. First, they demonstrate that any efforts to reduce health care costs must be directed at the high users, simply because they

Table 3.2

Lifestyle and Self-Inflicted Diseases

Lifestyle	Self-Inflicted Diseases
Obesity	Hypertension, diabetes, heart disease, varicose veins
Alcohol abuse	Cirrhosis of the liver, encephalopathy, Fetal Alcohol Syndrome
Cigarette smoking	Emphysema, chronic bronchitis, lung cancer, coronary artery disease
Drug abuse	Suicide, homicide, overdose, malnutrition, infectious diseases
High fat intake	Arteriosclerosis, diabetes, coronary artery disease
Low-fiber diet	Colorectal cancer
Sedentary lifestyle	Coronary artery disease, hypertension
Failure to wear seat belts	Increased incidence of severe injury and death
Sexual promiscuity	STDs, AIDS, cervical cancer

Source: Adapted from Leichter (1991:77).

consume such a large proportion of the resources. Any significant cost savings must come from these people, not the large majority that collectively uses very little. Berk and Monheit note that "There are serious limitations to the effectiveness of any cost-containment strategies that focus on the 90 percent of the population that collectively accounts for only one-third of the total U.S. health care spending." Second, the data demonstrate that considerable redistribution of societal resources is necessary if these individuals, many of whom are poor, are able to obtain the health services they need. Third, they raise serious questions concerning the extent to which society can afford to support individuals who knowingly engage

Table 3.3

Causes of Death in the United States, 2000

Cause	Estimated Number of Deaths	Percentage of Total Deaths
Tobacco	435,000	18.1
Diet/activity patterns	400,000	16.6
Alcohol	85,000	3.5
Microbial agents	75,000	3.1
Toxic agents	55,000	2.3
Motor vehicles	43,000	1.8
Firearms	29,000	1.2
Sexual behavior	20,000	0.9
Illicit use of drugs	17,000	0.7
Total	1,159,000	48.2

Source: Mokdad et al. 2004.

in high-risk behavior. This is a particularly salient issue when these needed services include long-term, expensive interventions such as intensive care and organ transplantation. A peripheral issue centers on the fact that with this knowledge, private insurers are able to selectively exclude from coverage groups and individuals that are likely to be in these high-risk categories based on their lifestyles. Without government regulations prohibiting this pattern, the low-risk, healthy groups become concentrated in the private sector whereas actual and potential high users must turn to the public sector.

Restoring the Concept of Individual Responsibility for Health

In Chapter 2, we argued that rationing needs to become more explicit and systematic, and nowhere is this more divisive than when medical resources are denied individuals because they have contributed to their own ill health. Moreover, the most difficult preventive measures are likely to be those in which the individual has prime responsibility. Any attempts by the government to intervene in lifestyle decisions are inherently controversial. Even relatively innocuous laws requiring motorcyclists to wear safety helmets have been attacked by some as a paternalistic. Despite the difficulties of addressing the issue of individual responsibility in a culture of individual rights, pressures emerging from the health care crisis necessitate a much closer look at (1) the role individuals play in contributing to their own health problems, (2) a shift of responsibility for health toward the individual, and (3) a return to the idea that individuals have an obligation to society to do those things that maximize their own health and thus reduce the burden on others who pay the bills.

Momentum for this reevaluation of personal responsibility comes from the mounting understanding of the costs of unhealthy behaviors and distaste at having to pay more for health care because of the bad habits of others. This demand for societal action in part reflects a desire for protection from the huge costs of calamities others bring upon themselves—in others words, it is a demand for fairness. The specter of unbounded increases in health care costs reflected in skyrocketing medical insurance premiums fuels the demand that people engaging in a high-risk or unhealthy behavior pay their own way. Because few people today pay fully for their own medical care, illness is a social expense. This means that people who try to take care of themselves are underwriting the costs incurred by those who fail to do so. As a result, there has been a call to shift the monetary burden to individuals who knowingly take the health risks, reflected in lower insurance premiums for nonsmokers, recommendations to raise the tax on alcoholic beverages, and corporate incentives for participation in physical fitness programs. Moreover, antiobesity programs are commencing in the United States, though it is doubtful they will soon go as far as the United Kingdom, where in 2003 the government announced a controversial plan to deny obese patients National Health Service care unless they lost weight.

> People who engage in high-risk behaviors contribute inequitably to escalating health care costs and, along with the very elderly, constitute the high users of medical care.

One of the central tenets of a liberal society is that there is no one conception of the good life; in other words, individuals have a right to live their lives as they desire, as long as they do not harm others. This value, when taken to its extreme, leads to the viewpoint that society cannot legitimately tell people how they ought to live. If people want to engage in behavior that is dangerous to their health, that is their business. One extension of this position is that society should not deny health care resources to people who contribute to or even cause their own ill health and that any such policy represents victim blaming. However, diseases of our era increasingly are the product of individual lifestyle choices. People who engage in high-risk behaviors contribute inequitably to escalating health care costs and, along with the very elderly, constitute the high users of medical care. More importantly, any efforts to prevent disease, improve population health, and constrain health costs require intervention in individual behavior and a renewed emphasis on individual responsibility for health. To argue otherwise in light of current disease patterns and medical evidence is to ignore reality.

The debate over the role of individual choice in determining personal health, although now intensifying, is far from new. According to Plato, individuals have a responsibility to live in a manner that prevents illness. Those who fail to do so have no claim on community resources for treatment. Likewise, the Greek physician Galen concluded that people who knowingly allow harm to come to their bodies and have the capacity to prevent it are morally culpable. This view of individual culpability for illness remained prevalent until the end of the nineteenth century. Although it is doubtful that the concept of individual responsibility for health was ever fully displaced, knowledge about the relationship between poor social conditions and disease and a resulting heightened social awareness shifted emphasis toward societal responsibility for public health. In the light of evidence that disease was caused largely by inadequate water and sewerage systems and by abhorrent working conditions over which individuals had little control, there emerged the view that only society, not the individual, had the means to overcome poverty and disease. Responsibility for disease prevention measures was placed on patients and their physicians, but public health programs proliferated to ameliorate unhealthy social conditions. Through the 1960s at least, individual responsibility for personal health was disparaged and those people who raised the issue were criticized as lacking a social conscience. Public incursions into matters of individual behavior were considered outside the legitimate sphere of government intervention.

In 1979, much debate followed publication of the Surgeon General's report *Healthy People*, which concluded that the foremost causes of modern illness lie in individual behavior and could be met most effectively through extensive changes in the lifestyles of many Americans. The tone of the report echoed John Knowles's earlier-cited admonition that the idea of a right to health should be "replaced by the idea of an individual moral obligation to preserve one's own health—a public duty, if you will." Two decades later, in his address to Congress unveiling the Health Security Act, President Clinton emphasized responsibility as his sixth principle: "In short, responsibility should apply to anybody who abuses the system and drives up the cost for honest, hard-working citizens. ... Responsibility also means changing some behaviors in this country that drive up our costs like crazy. And without changing it, we'll never have the system we ought to have."

This individual-responsibility model is in direct conflict with the social-responsibility model, under which an individual is not held personally accountable for the results of his or her actions. It must always be the fault of someone or something else (for example, genetics). Whereas the social model recoils from placing blame on the person, the individual model makes explicit the goal of assigning personal responsibility. The social model is reflected in the proclivity of Americans to avoid personal responsibility by shifting the blame to others, often business or government. Clear illustrations of this are lawsuits by smokers against cigarette manufacturers and obese people against fast-food chains. It has been said that people who overeat used to be called gluttons, but now they are called victims.

In contrast, under a personal-responsibility model, when the condition requiring care is predictable and avertable and the person behaves in a manner so as to incur the condition, it might be termed "deserved." Although it seems indecent to let someone suffer or die for lack of easily available treatment, when economic constraints make the provision of all health needs impossible, "even those who accept the ideal of freedom may endorse some restrictions on choice to correct for inevitable distortions of judgment," as noted by George Sher.

There is no shortage of critics who view moves toward targeting individual behavior as regressive and dangerous and who are especially hostile to any social sanctions imposed on individuals who refuse to change their risky ways. Faith Fitzgerald, for instance, warns against a zealotry about rationing by lifestyle where "we can blame patients for their illnesses and deny them both our compassion and our services. The thrust toward rationing of health care is making the association between vice and disease a public policy." Ruth Chadwick contends that society's "notion of deserving" is not an appropriate factor for allocating health care resources and argues that the problem with the idea of individual responsibility for health is that it gives insignificant weight to social causes of disease and to the context within which individual choices are made. Victim blaming, according to Chadwick, is especially unfair because much unhealthy behavior stems from society itself or from uncontrollable causes. Another argument against individual responsibility for ill health is that any system designed to enforce individual responsibility's role in allocation is unworkable because there is no sharp line between those people who take unreasonable health risks and those who do not, since we all take some risks.

Although the fervent reaction against individual responsibility for health is not surprising, rewarding unhealthy behaviors by guaranteeing medical interventions to ameliorate the problems individuals cause reinforces harmful routines. Instead of enabling unhealthy behavior, we ought to make it socially and culturally unacceptable. Our society has gone too far in maximizing individual rights at the expense of personal responsibility. There needs to be restoration of a balance that is now absent and restrictions on risky individual behaviors, because limiting liberties to promote the public health is to promote a common good, not a private or paternalistic one. As Dan Beauchamp states, "The American insistence on absolute autonomy has a kind of mystic quality that badly needs deflating" if we are to serve the collective interests.

> Rewarding unhealthy behaviors by guaranteeing medical interventions to ameliorate the problems individuals cause reinforces harmful routines.

In order to control health care costs, then, we must set reasonable boundaries on the rights to health care and restate the notion of individual responsibility for health. Every right ought to carry with it a corresponding obligation to those upon whom the claim is levied. This is especially relevant in attempts to link allocation and rationing criteria to individual lifestyle choices. In order to claim societal health resources, a person should be expected to act responsibly and not unduly contribute to the risk of ill health. Although people may have a right to design their own lifestyle, if they choose to engage in practices and behaviors that put them at high risk, they should be prepared to relinquish their claim on societal health care resources. By failing to balance rights with responsibilities, they surrender positive extensions of those rights.

The starting point for reducing unhealthy and unsafe personal behavior is education, and that education should come before habits are formed, preferably early in youth. Health education, however, has received little support under our dominant medical model, with less than 1 percent of total health expenditures so allocated. Also, though education is the most acceptable means of promoting healthy personal lifestyles, it alone is unlikely to drastically alter individual behaviors that enjoy broad attraction to many people. Appeals to the individual's own future health as well as to more-general social goals have failed to avert the expenditure of a large proportion of the health care budget on conditions and diseases that are preventable. Just go to any American all-you-can-eat restaurant for evidence of this.

> Although people may have a right to design their own lifestyle, if they choose to engage in practices and behaviors that put them at high risk, they should be prepared to relinquish their claim on societal health care resources.

Another option short of rationing medicine by lifestyle is to make those who engage in high-risk activities contribute more to the health care budget. "Sin taxes" have become an attractive source of general revenue over and above their use in recouping excess costs linked to unhealthy behavior, and their inclusion in the Clinton Health Security Act was among the proposal's most popular aspects. They are made more attractive because they are viewed as taxing undesirable behavior as well as compensating for external costs caused by people indulging in it. For instance, it is estimated that a 1 cent per twelve-ounce soft drink tax would generate $1.5 billion annually. The public furor over the idea of taxing junk food, for example, the "Twinkie tax," to combat obesity, however, shows that any attempt by government to influence eating behavior will be viewed as heavy-handed intrusion on the freedom to live as one pleases, as suggested by Radley Balko, who argues that "Nutrition activists are agitating for a panoply of initiatives that would bring the government between you and your waistline."

Actions by schoolboards to ban snacks and soda from school campuses, calls for a "fat tax" on high-calorie foods, and menu-labeling legislation are the wrong way to fight obesity, according to Balko. If we "Give Americans moral, financial, and personal responsibility for their own health, obesity will no longer be a public matter but a private one."

It has been suggested that under "a rebalanced health care system" it would be possible to fund health care mainly through taxes on commodities that contribute to poor health. In addition to raising revenues, another goal of such taxes is to increase the costs of these commodities and thus reduce consumption. It is estimated that for every 10 percent increase in the price of cigarettes, adult consumption decreases by 4 percent. Another proposal that is common overseas is to tax alcohol heavily: a $2 per ounce tax on alcohol translates to $13 on a six-pack of beer, $12 on a 750 ml bottle of wine, and $40 on a 750 ml bottle of 100-proof liquor. Although such a tax is likely to shrink alcohol usage and provide revenue in the short run, given the political influence of the alcohol industry and the drinking public, it is not politically feasible.

Moreover, though the sin tax strategy is intuitively attractive, except for tobacco and alcohol, its implementation is problematic. To be fair, such schemes should include all products or behaviors that lead to ill health, such as skiing, junk food, motorcycles, contact sports, and other risky activities. The problem is that such a list is endless and our understanding of the scientific basis of health and disease and the relative contributions of individual behaviors changes over time. Furthermore, society's view of acceptable and unacceptable actions clouds the objectivity in determining what might be taxed. A final problem with taxing unhealthy behavior is that many risky behaviors are illegal. Taxing alcohol and cigarettes but not marijuana, cocaine, heroin, or other substances is counterproductive. Perhaps this supports the case for legalizing these drugs and taxing them at rates commensurate with their health costs, but this seems unlikely to occur. The same can be said for prostitution and other activities that increase the risk and thus the health costs of promiscuous sex. Equitable implementation of taxing health-risk behaviors is not feasible or easily enforceable.

Another option is to increase the premiums paid into the health system by those individuals who engage in high-risk behaviors. Again, though this approach seems

> Many individuals at highest risk are not covered by the private insurance system and thus not influenced by higher premiums.

logical and is intuitively more fair than rationing, like taxation it is inherently selective in nature and has tended to focus on smoking, even though alcohol use, obesity, and a sedentary lifestyle are more likely to increase costs for the average person. Additionally, many individuals at highest risk are not covered by the private insurance system and thus not influenced by higher premiums. Although increased premiums for unhealthy behaviors enjoy wide public support and provide the appearance of fairness, they too fail to deliver needed incentives for individual responsibility.

Rationing by Lifestyle

Although serious efforts to decrease unhealthy behavior make good sense and preventing the government from interfering with individual choice does not, ultimately individuals who persist in such lifestyles should be denied certain types of health care. Although many ethicists and social commentators condemn such targeted rationing, the coming health care crisis and the concentration of health spending noted here demands contemplation that individuals who harm themselves be denied expensive medical technologies that are in scarce supply. As Tristram Engelhardt concludes: "It will also be morally acceptable for society, if it pursues expensive lifesaving treatment, to exclude persons who through their own choices increase the cost of care. ... There is no invidious discrimination against persons in setting limits to coverage or in precluding coverage if the costs are increased through free choice." This said, questions abound as to how lifestyle criteria should be expressly entered into the rationing equation and who is responsible for establishing the criteria.

As individuals come to pay larger amounts in out-of-pocket costs or insurance premiums, the issue of individual responsibility will intensify. Individuals who try to take care of themselves will realize that they are paying the costs of the deleterious behavior of a minority of citizens who use a disproportionate amount of health care. At present, this cost shifting is not transparent, because the tab is largely borne by third-party payers. With a severe tightening up of Medicare and Medicaid spending and the increased use of managed care, the extent of the burden on the health system by individuals who live unhealthy lifestyles will become more apparent. Already, many medical personnel are aware of the large proportion of their time devoted to individuals who refuse to protect their health, and they "find it a particular affront that anyone would deliberately risk it," as Einer Elhauge noted. Although it is politically incorrect to call for such rationing, this is the direction in which we must move.

If we are serious about controlling the health cost explosion, we must ration resources away from the high users. Directly or indirectly, rationing will reduce the medical resources going to individuals who engage in high-risk behaviors. The remaining question is whether to make individual behavior an explicit basis upon which to deny health care. Excluding those situations where such individuals will be denied treatment because they are poorer medical risks, are less compliant, or have less-optimistic prognoses than individuals with healthy lifestyles, given equal need and equal prognosis, should lifestyle count? Even though medical ethics rightly excludes the medical community itself from considering lifestyle per se, public policy can and should make distinctions. Despite the difficulties and the problems raised by the critics, explicit policies that ration high-cost medical interventions away from individuals who have clearly contributed to or caused their ill health are the fairest route. Although understandably problematic, we need to make inroads into the escalating costs of caring for high users. Although one result of such rationing might be to save significant resources, the primary goal is to put all citizens on notice that the assumption of unlimited medical support is no longer assured for those

Box 3.2
A Case for Concern

Although extreme cases do not always make good policy, we can't ignore them in framing policy responses to health problems. As such, the case of forty-two-year-old Patrick Duel raises the point of how much we can afford to pay to treat self-inflicted health conditions. Mr. Duel weighed 1,072 pounds when he checked into the hospital in June 2004 dying of heart failure. His doctor recommended gastric bypass surgery, but his heart problems, complicated by diabetes and other health conditions caused by his obesity, prevented this. Instead, he was admitted to the hospital where he spent three months on a 1,200 calorie-a-day diet and exercise regime and lost 420 pounds. Stomach surgery was performed in October, and he was due from release from the hospital on January 22, 2005. Mr. Duel relies totally on Medicare and Medicaid to pay all his health care bills, which continue to mount. Although he represents an extreme high user, Mr. Duel is not alone in his need for massive health care resources that could be used much more effectively elsewhere.

people who refuse to take responsibility for their own health.

Under this policy, all people, no matter what their lifestyle, should have access to a basic package of health care, which includes primary care and a limited range of acute and chronic care. Other interventions, such as organ transplantation, kidney dialysis, and intensive care, should be provided only after resources are available to meet the basic needs of all citizens. We need to draw lines somewhere. A good place to start is to reduce funding for those procedures that are primarily used to rescue people from the results of their own behavior. Such a system would be dependent on a shift from demand-side price rationing to supply-side non-price rationing because under the current open-ended system, a David Crosby or Evel Knievel can always get their transplant because it is rationed by price. This transformation in effect would move our rationing policy toward those found in other democracies where traditionally there has been much greater emphasis on individual responsibility and collective good.

Age as a Consideration in Rationing

We turn now to the second of our two groups of high users of health care. Despite its controversy, age rationing is essential if we are to create a sustainable health care system. All one has to do is just stand back and look at the figures. At present, over 45 percent of health care resources go to the approximately 12.7 percent of the population that is sixty-five years of age or older. Americans who turned sixty-five in 1994 can expect to receive on average about $200,000 worth of health care before they die, with approximately one-third of that spent in the last year of life. Moreover, within this over-sixty-five grouping, the small fraction that is over age eighty accounts for many times the average

> At present, over 45 percent of health care resources go to the approximately 12.7 percent of the population that is sixty-five years of age or older.

expenditure of the over-sixty-five cohort. Given these spending inequities, the health care trends in the aging of the population are most troubling. With the retirement of the baby boomers in the coming decades, unless something is done to change this spending pattern, these burgeoning cohorts will consume an even larger proportion of health care spending, thus sucking in even greater resources from other areas. Simply put, we cannot rein in health care costs without using age as a criterion in rationing, simply because the elderly are the prime users of technologies that increase the costs of medicine.

Paradoxically, age is already a consideration in the delivery of health care in that we give universal coverage to most of those over sixty-five while ignoring other age groups completely. We ration health care in favor of the elderly. Per capita government spending for the elderly in 2001 was $4,360, compared to $258 for children. Overall, there is a seventeen-to-one ratio of total public spending for the health care of the elderly compared to that of children, a difference that will grow considerably when the Medicare prescription drug benefit is fully implemented. Although practically we can understand this as the result of political pressures from those who vote in the largest numbers and percentage, it is hard to justify morally. Moreover, as a matter of social policy, this spending would seem to favor those whose economically productive lives are largely over at the expense of younger workers whom the economy relies on for its fruits. Working America now supports two groups that are morally important but marginal to the economy: those on welfare (Medicaid) and the elderly (Medicare and Medicaid). At some point in the near future, this is bound to become an explosive issue as workers are asked to increase their taxes substantially to meet the health needs of a growing elderly population.

Although as a concept age rationing is currently in violation of federal law, age must be included as *one* factor in the delivery of health care. Every religion, every culture, every civilization differentiates between a premature death and death after a long life. Society owes a greater moral duty to a ten-year-old with her or his whole life ahead than to a ninety-year-old, no matter how healthy the latter might be. We should not differentiate the health care delivered between men or women or on the basis of race, ethnicity, or geography, but unlike those distinctions, age is an equal-opportunity status. We all get older year after year in a marvelously egalitarian way. Age is not a static group, but rather a state that we all go through, thus shifting limited resources from the elderly to the young is essential. Norman Daniels is correct when he notes that it is a mistake to think of the elderly as a competing group instead of as citizens at a different stage of life. He introduces the prudential life span account in which distribution of resources between different age groups is viewed as a problem of prudential reasoning for an individual regarding how to distribute resources over the different stages of his or her life. The question is not what generation gets what, but at what stage of life can we best spend limited resources and for what. Rationing policy that considers age is not age discrimination, it's a commonsense answer to the question of who should get limited resources.

The maldistribution of health resources in favor of the elderly will escalate in part because more-intensive technologies and drug options continually increase the range of potential interventions and thus the relative costs of high users. More important, however, is the quantity of health resources required by an aging population. It is a fact of life that the older we become, the more health resources we consume. Because of the higher incidence of illness among the elderly, particularly of costly, chronic diseases, people over age sixty-five enter the hospital twice as often as younger people, and they stay longer. Average per capita expenditure is approximately four times higher for the elderly than the nonelderly, and, more importantly, the rate of increase in such spending for the elderly is nearly three times that of the nonelderly. Ironically, because of medical improvements and technologies that prolong life, chronic disease requiring frequent medical care has become an increasing drain on scarce medical resources. People who in earlier times would have died of one illness are often kept alive to suffer long-term decline in quality of life. However, the demand for such intervention will continue to increase as the population ages. Furthermore, because of the concurrence of multiple and often chronic conditions, the cost of prolonging life at older ages is higher than at younger ones, increasingly so since the introduction of antibiotics reduced the incidence of death from illnesses such as pneumonia.

The elderly use more acute care, are hospitalized about twice as often, stay longer in hospitals, and are much more likely to be readmitted to the hospital. Nearly half (47 percent) of all ICU patients are over age sixty-five, which means 12.7 percent of the population consumes nearly one-half of the nation's critical care resources. The cost of ICU care for a patient over age sixty-five is three to five times more per day than the cost of resources utilized for the average acute-care admission. Baby boomers are just entering the fifty-five to sixty-four age group, where, according to PricewaterhouseCoopers, inpatient medical days per thousand are 58 percent higher than in the forty-five to fifty-four age group and 121 percent higher than in the thirty-five to forty-four age group. Moreover, it is estimated by the Clinical Advisory Board that current baby boomers could outlive today's elderly by seven to fifteen years, thus requiring a doubling of ICU care over the next fifteen years. According to a study by James Fries et al., approximately four-fifths of people over sixty-five have one or more chronic conditions and the costs of these conditions are often overlooked. Almost 80 percent of health care costs currently result from chronic conditions that occur between the age of fifty-five and the end of life. Moreover, three of every four deaths in the United States come as a result of a degenerative disease, usually in advanced age. As the numbers of elderly rise, their increased costs for medical services will consume a larger and larger share of societal health care budgets. We can spend endless amounts of our scarce national resources on arthritis, hypertension and heart disease, orthopedic conditions (osteoporosis), hearing or vision impairment, and sinusitis. With 20 percent of those over the age of eighty-five

> Even if improved lifestyles and medical technologies are successful in reducing the major causes of premature death, we will be left with a rapidly growing elderly population whose additional years of life may be dominated by nonfatal but highly debilitating conditions such as arthritis, osteoporosis, and Alzheimer's disease.

in nursing homes, where will we get the resources to warehouse those aging bodies?

Furthermore, advances in medical treatment allow elderly people who are frail and suffer from fatal degenerative diseases to survive longer after the onset of the disease than in the past. The result is that age-specific morbidity and disability rates and their duration have increased exponentially. As S. Jay Olshansky et al. note, "Even if rates of morbidity and disability remain constant, the number of people surviving with conditions of frailty will expand because of the rapid growth in the size of the elderly population resulting from population aging and declining old-age mortality." Even if improved lifestyles and medical technologies are successful in reducing the major causes of premature death, we will be left with a rapidly growing elderly population whose additional years of life may be dominated by nonfatal but highly debilitating conditions such as arthritis, osteoporosis, and Alzheimer's disease. The result could be longer life but worsening health, thus an actual decline in active life expectancy. Under these circumstances, health care becomes Sisyphean, where we conquer one disease only to throw ourselves into the arms of another disease as we attempt to fill this fiscal black hole by using resources that are desperately needed by other generations.

The aging of the population in itself is not the major threat. Many other countries provide universal coverage for considerably older populations at lower aggregate cost. What is potentially catastrophic is the combination of an aging population and a health care system where there are no formalized constraints on the amount of resources devoted to high-technology intervention for the elderly. As noted by Daniel Callahan, although we are likely to muddle along for several decades until the problem becomes unendurable, the trend in heavy investment in the elderly must be moderated well before that time. Ivan Illich is outspoken on this matter:

> They [the aged] have been trained to experience urgent needs that no level of *relative* privilege can possibly satisfy. The more tax money that is spent to bolster their frailty, the keener is their awareness of decay. At the same time, their ability to take care of themselves has withered, as social arrangements allowing them to exercise autonomy have practically disappeared.

Because there is nothing that can be done to stem the aging population, the only feasible option is to drastically scale down our expectations and delimit technological interventions beyond a reasonable point, in other words, to ration care for the elderly.

As financial and ethical pressures mount, the right to death with dignity should be transformed into an expectation and eventually into an obligation, even though this development will create enormous stress for patients and their families, health professionals, and government. Although this development is foreign to our cultural values, is inevitable that at some point even well-insured elderly can no longer expect all the care that might do them some good. Unless we start to change expectations now, our children are going to wake up someday and see how badly we screwed things up. As Paul Menzel states, "What is clear is that people of integrity, appreciating all the ages they might live into, will not hide their heads in the sand about what the real costs of life-saving are, including later health-care expenses and added years of pension benefits. There's seldom a free lunch, and life-saving care in old age is certainly not one of them."

> As financial and ethical pressures mount, the right to death with dignity should be transformed into an expectation and eventually into an obligation, even though this development will create enormous stress for patients and their families, health professionals, and government.

The most common argument against considering age in health care decisions is that such rationing amounts to age discrimination and is especially unfair because of the past contributions made to society by the elderly. In other words, society owes the elderly their just rewards. In contrast, the "fair innings" argument contends that it is just that those people who have already had more than

their fair share of life and its delights should not be preferred to the younger person who has not been so favored.
Otherwise stated, it is unfair to deny the young the
opportunity to become old while allowing those who are
already old to become older. Another argument against
considering age in rationing is the Kantian view that society must value people not merely as means to productive
or efficient output but as ends in themselves. Critics also
reject economic arguments that greater savings are made
from denying care to the old because younger people are
relatively more productive to society, that more life-years
are gained by giving preference to younger people, or
that the elderly, on average, consume more health care
resources. Moreover, the view that the elderly are less
able to benefit from treatment is countered by those who
reject chronological age as a meaningful gauge of benefit
and argue that all patients should be assessed for treatment on the basis of their physiology alone.

Others argue that rationing itself is the problem and
the harm is compounded by using age as a criterion.
Patricia Blanchette, for example, contends that care must
be appropriate, not rationed, and concludes that under-
rationing is easy to bait into an intergenerational contest,
pitting the costs of providing increasingly sophisticated
care to younger patients against the costs of caring for
the nation's elders. In contrast, others agree with our view
that age is *one* legitimate and necessary consideration
in rationing. Alan Williams suggests that we should not
object to age being a criteria used in the prioritization of
health care, because the alternative is too outrageous to
contemplate—namely, that we expect the young to make
large sacrifices so that the elderly can enjoy small benefits.
Also, he states that "This vain pursuit of immortality is

dangerous for elderly people: taken to its logical conclusion it implies that no one should be allowed to die
until everything possible has been done. That means not
simply that we shall die in a hospital but that we shall
die in intensive care." Likewise, Anthony Shaw concludes
that other things being equal, there is a greater duty to
use our scarce resources to prolong the lives of younger
than older people, though he notes that chronological
age should be a weighing factor in rationing decisions,
but not an absolute bar to which we agree.

No one has had more impact on the age-rationing
debate than Daniel Callahan. He argues that even with
relatively ample resources, there will be better ways in the
future to spend our money than on indefinitely extending
the life of the elderly. According to Callahan, a natural life
span is one in which life's possibilities have on the whole
been achieved and after which death may be understood
as a sad, but nonetheless relatively acceptable event. To
this end, we must abandon the notion that we should try
endlessly through medical progress to revise old age and
instead accept aging as a part of life, not just another medical obstacle to overcome. An extension of this argument
is Dan Brock's call for "weak age rationing," under which
greater weight is given to the claims on social resources
for life-sustaining care up to, as opposed to beyond, the
normal life span. A similar argument is based on the
premise that old age and death are in the natural order
and, like any other inevitability, they must be accepted,
not resisted at all costs.

Clearly we should never abandon the elderly (we will
all be there someday), and certainly we owe a high duty
of care to people whatever their age. But there are certain
high-cost or high-technology procedures that must be

limited by age. In an informal and haphazard way, we already do this. Strong evidence exists that many health professionals provide differential treatment for elderly patients regardless of comparable diagnoses, prognoses, or other potentially explanatory factors. Marshall Kapp, for instance, contends that through covert implicit rationing, age-based rationing de facto takes place every day on the basis of individual bedside decisions and actions by physicians and nurses regarding individual patients. Would it not be more honest and fair to formalize this situation? We strongly endorse the views of Larry Churchill when he observes: "We should encourage a prudent system that does not create an expectation of automatic use, and that curtails the availability of very expensive, marginally effective life-extending technologies for the elderly." The first part of this challenge is to reevaluate the goals of medicine and ask if life extension beyond a certain point is either a valid social or medical goal. *The Hastings Center Report* study on the goals of medicine must start our dialogue:

> An appropriate aim first and foremost is to reduce premature death in populations generally and individuals particularly. A secondary purpose is to care appropriately for those whose death would no longer be considered premature, but who could nonetheless benefit from medical treatment. ... the primary duty of medicine and health care systems [should be] to help the young become old, and then, that accomplished, to help those who are old live out the remainder of their lives in dignity and comfort.

Dignity and comfort does not, of course, require us to do everything that is technologically possible to prolong life. Not surprisingly, using age as a factor in rationing has been widely condemned in the United States, though in countries such as the United Kingdom old age "is a criterion for rationing health resources and it occurs at all levels of the National Health Service," as noted by Bradley Williams.

Whatever one's view on whether the elderly are getting their fair share of the health budget or if they ought to get less than younger people because they have had their "fair innings" (or fair share earlier in life), there is no denying that the aging population is a major problem for the distribution of health care resources and, in fact, in the redistribution of all societal resources. It is also clear that the problem will get progressively worse and that existing priorities in health policy are not only not sufficient, but also counterproductive. Any debate over setting limits to medical technologies and rationing health care must address the intergenerational redistribution of resources as well as the implications of any policy changes for the elderly. It is likely that as the issues raised here become fathomed by the current younger generations (especially those people now under thirty), a form of intergenerational warfare will ensue. Unfortunately, the battle lines are becoming increasingly intransigent as the crisis looms and the stakes heighten.

―――――

What we see in the attacks on rationing by age and by lifestyle are not-so-subtle attacks on explicit rationing per se because the critics realize that any systematic rationing must limit the kind of health care services most heavily used by these two groups. They know that taking age and lifestyle factors out of the rationing equation effectively guts it. It makes little sense to consider rationing without targeting high users. The very fact that the elderly and risk takers are disproportionately heavy health care users requires that attention be directed to them. Age and individual behavior must be considered as but two of many factors in any attempts to constrain health care spending, but they must in any case be addressed.

Chapter 4
Controlling Medical Technology

Although technological medicine has expanded in all
Western nations, a unique set of values, practices, and
structures in the United States has exaggerated the forces
driving the diffusion of technology.[1] America has made a
Faustian bargain with its medical technology. Despite the
fact that much more national health could be produced
by expanding coverage of the uninsured or improving
the health delivery system, we constantly produce new
and often marginal technologies while ignoring other
more health-producing opportunities. We automatically
assume that a new technology is health producing without analysis or any consideration of opportunity costs.
Mesmerized by technology, we are following an unsustainable path that misallocates limited health resources
and values marginal advances for the insured over basic
coverage of the uninsured. A combination of faith in
technology to provide health care, a powerful medical research industry, and an incentive structure that
rewards individualized medicine and innovation assures
dominance of the supply state. In contrast, those nations

[1] Jacobs terms this distinctive U.S. commitment to expand the supply of
technologically sophisticated medicine the "American supply state" and
contrasts it with the higher priority put on access to health care in other
nations (1995:143).

that emphasize universal access have by necessity limited development and diffusion of medical technologies by constraining facility development, emphasizing primary care physicians over specialists, and exercising governmental planning authority. These nations have put medical technology in a much more balanced perspective.

Control of the unbridled proliferation of medical technology must be a high priority, even if it means some individuals will be denied potential lifesaving innovations. In light of the current value system and incentive structure and the unwillingness to institute some form of global budgeting, however, this will require not only major structural changes, but also an intensified resolve to grasp the severity of the problems facing us. Public policy must prevent America's love of technology from completely unbalancing its health care system. Technology is important, but it cannot continue to dominate other important needs. Unless we adopt a realistic view of the deleterious influence of the supply-state dominance, universal access and cost control will continue to be elusive.

> We spend hundreds of billions of dollars on new technologies and virtually nothing on better managing what we already have.

We accept and appreciate the role of medical technology in improving the health of America. It is the total lack of balance, the blind assumption that medical research and technology are the best (almost the only) way to improve the health of the nation that is disturbing. We spend hundreds of billions of dollars on new technologies and virtually nothing on better managing what we already have. We search for "technological immorality" for ourselves while our neighbor has serious but easily resolved medical needs that go unmet.

The explosion of new medical technologies over the past several decades has been one of the most important drivers of health care spending growth, if not the most important. These innovations can improve care but tend to cost more than older forms of treatment. Even taken individually, the availability of specific technologies is associated with sizable spending growth. Laurence Baker et al. analyzed the relationship between the supply of new technologies in diagnostic imaging, cardiac, cancer, and newborn care and found that increases in the supply of technology tend to be related to higher usage and spending on the service in question. In some cases increases in availability appear to be associated with new applications rather than substitution for other services. We are spending more and more, often for less and less. As Baker notes, "For diagnostic imaging, for both the commercial and Medicare plans, more availability of freestanding MRI facilities is associated with a higher number of outpatient MRI procedures per population and higher spending on outpatient MRI. ... a one unit increase in the number of freestanding MRI units per million people is associated with an increase of about $32,900 per million beneficiaries per month, or approximately $395,000 per year."

Virtually all scholars agree that the biomedical revolution relentlessly drives up health care spending. Moreover, this cost-increasing effect of medical technology is not an aberration, because scientific revolutions always increase total spending. Kenneth Thorpe et al., for example, found that a small number of medical conditions were associated with much of the increase in health care spending between 1987 and 2000, with the top fifteen conditions accounting for approximately half of the overall growth in spending. For some of

Box 4.1
The Cost of Technology

The price tag for treating cancer patients with new biotech drugs has increased 500-fold in the last decade. Ten years ago, doctors could extend the life of a patient by an average 11.5 months using a combination of drugs that cost $500 in today's dollars. Now, new medicines can extend survival to 22.5 months but at a cost of $250,000, not including pharmacy markups, salaries for doctors and nurses, and the cost of infusing the drugs into patients in the hospital. That kind of cost increase is unsustainable. "Sooner or later the bubble is going to pop," according to Memorial Sloan-Kettering cancer doctor Leonard Saltz . How many costly cancer drugs can society afford to stack on top of one another? "Absent a thoughtful national discussion, the answer is none," says Michael A. Friedman, chief executive of City of Hope cancer center in Los Angeles. The rising costs are "utterly insupportable" and we will "quickly run out of resources, leading to de facto rationing."

— Matthew Herper, "Cancer's Cost Crisis," *Forbes*, June 8, 2004

these conditions, most of the increase was associated with increased treated prevalence, which either may reflect improvements in medical technology that allow expanded treatment of a particular condition or changes in the diagnosis or reporting of disease.

We don't give up an inch of moral high ground here, for the excess and duplication of medical technology is realistically harming many more people than if it were expanded thoughtfully. If we step back from the bedside and the insatiable demands of autonomy, we see what every other developed country sees: that medical technology can be an encumbrance unless thoughtfully developed and defused. Even though it is likely that the bulk of health care spending on new technologies fails to produce higher quality, it is also likely that some new technologies do produce value for patients.[2]

The problem of priority setting will become more acute in the coming decade because we are likely to see the rapid proliferation of costly "last chance" therapies: technologies that represent the last chance at prolonging life for individuals, are very expensive, and typically yield what might be judged marginal benefits relative to costs. Is society or a health plan obligated to provide them? Leonard Fleck examines three examples that have achieved media prominence: the totally implantable artificial heart (estimated 350,000 procedures per year, with an average of five extra years of life expectancy at a cost of $52 billion overall); the left ventricular assist device (200,000 procedures annually with a survival rate of one to two years); and Herceptin, a drug for women with metastasized breast cancer (prescribed to 12,000 women each year at a likely cost of $70,000 per case with average gain in life expectancy of five months, translating to a cost per life-year saved of about $168,000). In each case, there is nothing else that can be offered these patients. Is a just and caring society morally obligated to provide access to this therapy at social expense? These represent examples of Callahan's "ragged edge problem." According to Fleck, "We can imagine 'compassionate' legislative mandates that would require Medicare and private insurance companies to cover these 'last chance' therapies. But would that be a good thing to do? Should we applaud such efforts as another incremental step on the road to

---

[2] Baker and associates (2003) conclude that policy efforts to assess and manage the availability of new technologies could benefit society in instances where the additional spending produced by new services is not associated with quality improvements, but they caution that higher spending need not be purely negative for society if the spending yields sufficient benefits.

health reform?" Like Fleck, our response to both questions is no, because these are only the first wave of many even more costly therapies and there is no morally or rationally obvious place to draw a line. Furthermore, they dramatically increase health costs for the already insured, thereby making it even more unlikely to meet the basic health needs of the uninsured. The ragged edge problem will not vanish and, as illustrated above, the costs are boundless. We can no longer escape the need to make explicit rationing decisions regarding such technologies, decisions that are bound to be very painful but necessary in a world of limits.

Inappropriate Use of Technology

America is in love with technology generally, and medical technology in particular. We seem to value it for itself and with little sense that it can be overbuilt, overused, inappropriately used, or even counterproductive to the health of America. *Inappropriate use of technology* is an umbrella term used by Seymour Perry to define the possible misapplication of technology under a variety of circumstances including "use of technology in ignorance or for a marginal benefit to the patient, use of technology in the absence of evidence of its value or in spite of the fact that conclusive studies have not been done." Inappropriate use of technology then goes beyond the medical judgments that can lead to applications that are of questionable value to a particular patient and rather addresses systemwide acceptance of technologies without proper criteria.

The high economic stakes in the health care industry ensure rapid diffusion of new technologies in the absence of public controls.

As noted earlier, the high economic stakes in the

health care industry ensure rapid diffusion of new technologies in the absence of public controls. As warned by the Radical Statistics Group in Britain decades ago, "The idea that market forces should determine medical need in the community is likely to lead to inappropriate care." The fee-for-service retrospective reimbursement system further distorts the market because it fails to provide any effective mechanisms to constrain these market forces. Instead, it creates an incentive structure that rewards overuse of technologies and invasive procedures. The result is that many of the interventions widely used by the medical profession, especially specialties and subspecialties that organize around each innovation, have never been subjected to objective scrutiny nor assessed as to either their contribution to health or their cost effectiveness, as noted by Irene Butter. Another consequence is the perpetuation of illogical, expensive, and potentially dangerous practices carried on in the name of modern medicine.

In no country is the evidence of a medical marketplace run amok more obvious than in the United States. Because hospitals must keep up with the latest developments in order to compete for patients in the marketplace, the proliferation of technologies is rapid. Although the proliferation of medical technology means that insured Americans have access to the latest innovations, in many cases the interventions are of unproven benefit and, in some cases, can be dangerous to the patient. Furthermore, the diffusion of unproven interventions consumes ever-larger proportions of health care resources, thus diverting resources from everything from universal access to beneficial treatments, primary care, and prevention. As a result, there has been considerable critical analysis of spending patterns on innovative therapy, particularly those relating to heart disease and cancer.

The most authoritative evidence on the overuse of health care technologies in the United States comes from the Center for the Evaluative Clinical Sciences (CECS) at Dartmouth Medical School. The results of their studies show an interesting outcome. Among people in the United States who died between 1999 and 2003, per capita spending varied by a factor of six among hospitals across the country. Average utilization and spending varied from state to state, from region to region within states, and from hospital to hospital within the same regions. Importantly, spending levels were not correlated with rates of illness in different parts of the country, but rather reflected how intensively but variably certain resources—acute-care hospital beds, specialist physician visits, tests, and other services—were used in the management of people who were very ill but could not be cured. This supply-sensitive care accounts for well over 50 percent of all Medicare spending. What is most profound is that the findings of this report demonstrate that for chronically ill Americans, receiving more services does not result in improved outcomes and, in fact, these patients might be worse off. These findings are supported by other studies as well.

> The evidence that outcomes and quality of care tend to be better in regions with low resource use and low care intensity has important policy implications. ... at the population level, more intensive use of supply-sensitive care—more frequent physician visits, hospitalizations, and stays in intensive care among the chronically ill—does not result in better health outcomes.

Where is the moral outrage at such statistics? How can the findings of these uncontradicted studies remain uncorrected for so long? Where is the moral outrage at these excesses in a country that has so much unmet need?

Furthermore, and especially because most Americans say they prefer to avoid a "high-tech" death, the report concludes that Medicare spending for the care of the chronically ill could be reduced by as much as 30 percent while improving quality, patient satisfaction, and outcomes. Moreover, the problem of overuse of technology is growing as care intensity increases, especially in those regions that are already at the high end of spending and utilization rates. It is not solely the American public driving this, but a medical culture and technological imperative that have no apparent limits.

A related study by CECS associates Wennberg et al. found that Medicare pays some California hospitals four times more than others with no gain in quality or patient satisfaction. The study found that eliminating Medicare overcare by improving hospital efficiency could have saved Medicare $1.7 billion over five years in Los Angeles alone. Additionally, in their study of elderly Medicare patients with acute myocardial infarction, Therese Stukel et al. conclude that routine use of more costly and invasive treatment strategies may not be associated with an overall population benefit and that efforts should focus on directing invasive clinical resources to patients with the greatest expected benefit. Similarly, Jonathan Skinner et al. found that regions with the largest spending increases were not the ones realizing improvements in survival of patients for acute myocardial infarction.

> Eliminating Medicare overcare by improving hospital efficiency could have saved Medicare $1.7 billion over five years in Los Angeles alone.

And, crucially, those factors yielding the greatest benefits to health were not the factors that drove up the costs.

One question is the extent to which we can generalize beyond the critically ill patients on which the Dartmouth project focuses. Does the huge excess in health care spending of the United States as compared to other countries pay off in heightened levels of population health? Here the evidence is clear: the answer is a resounding no. The United States consistently rates below the top twenty nations, despite outspending many of them by almost a two to one ratio. A recent study by Lindsey Tanner, for example, found that the United States ranked near the bottom of industrialized nations for the survival rates of newborns, despite high spending on neonatal medicine: only Latvia had a lower rate. At the same time, other studies found that Americans aged fifty-five to sixty-four are much sicker than their British counterparts, even though the United States spends twice as much per person on health care, and that Canadians are healthier than their U.S. counterparts on almost every measure of health. Despite massive spending, Americans have higher rates of diabetes, hypertension, heart disease, stroke, lung disease, and cancer. But still we continue to spend ever more on medical technologies in search of a health care grail.

This captivation with technological fixes is reflected in the periodical emergence of breakthroughs in medical research that promise all manner of benefits. In the 1960s, for instance, Congress was told by scientists that if we declared a war on cancer and poured in research funding, cancer would be beaten. Similarly, in the 1960s and 1970s, Congress was promised a totally implantable and affordable artificial heart in a decade if funds were forthcoming. Then, in the 1980s, groundbreaking work in genetics and biotechnology was translated into highly enthusiastic predictions. Gene therapy, we were told, would revolutionize medicine, but even the more modest gene-therapy forecasts have yet to be realized, with signal projects often cut short because of safety concerns, even scandal. The same holds true for promises of AIDS researchers in the mid-1980s, some of whom contended that with enough research funds we would have an effective vaccine by 1990. Technology in America constantly overpromises, yet no one holds anyone accountable. In the United States particularly, a technological-fix mentality dominates, with elusive hopes of illusionary solutions attracting capital—and Congress. The most recent of these promises is stem-cell research.

We do not deny that medical science has made impressive technical advances, advances that at times immeasurably help individual patients and often exceed expectations, but promises of these big-science approaches have been routinely unmet. Even in the best of circumstances, stem-cell research is unlikely to deliver all the goods boosters now suggest: reversing paralysis, growing new organs, conquering diabetes and cancer, reversing the effects of neurodegenerative diseases such as Alzheimer's and Parkinson's, repairing heart-attack damage, restoring eyesight, creating neural tissues programmed to repair spinal cord injuries, growing full-thickness skin wherever burns have destroyed it. Importantly, as hyperbole raises false hopes it diverts resources that could better be used for preventive medicine and public-health promotion, where gains are likely to be more impressive overall.

Additionally, these new intervention possibilities come at a time when we can no longer afford to commit huge amounts of social resources without substantial evidence of likely success. Clearly, we must allocate resources to those areas most likely to contribute most efficiently to health. To date, cost-benefit projections of stem-cell research applications have been vague, perhaps understandably so at this early stage of development, but this has not stopped proponents from promising much. As noted earlier, however, the history of even modest medical innovations has been to escalate costs significantly, and we have little reason to believe that the results of stem-cell research would be any different, particularly if we are wrong and it fulfills all the promises now made. Although high cost is not reason enough to impede diffusion of potentially useful techniques, it must be a factor, however alien to our professed values; full policy analysis is not possible otherwise.

As noted above, the story of gene therapy is a cogent example of the overpromise of medical progress. Gene therapy experiments began in humans in 1990 with much fanfare. At the five-year mark, the National Institutes of Health issued a report showing that the first 600 people in the first 100 trials had not enjoyed any health benefits from the interventions. Clinical trials during the next five years were similarly disappointing, yet many still acclaim gene therapy. This is reflected in assertive, bold headlines such as "Rebecca Lilly's Brain Tumor Has Come Back for the Third Time: Can Gene Therapy Save Her Life?", which suggests to readers that gene therapy was already a standard of care (even though the hype was never substantiated in accompanying texts). And, the bioethics discussions similarly mulishly ignored the accumulating negative data.

Health Technology Assessment (HTA)

Thomas Bodenheimer suggests that controlling costs while preserving quality requires a multifaceted approach. In addition to strengthening primary care and disease management programs and reducing inappropriate care, medical errors, and the use of hospital and emergency departments by high-cost patients, we need the diffusion of effective technology assessment. The history of health technology assessment (HTA) has been an inconsistent and controversial one. It has been characterized by strong opposition from interests that see it as a threat to their autonomy and by criticism by those who feel it has failed to accomplish the objective of critical assessment, and thus failed to stem the dissemination of questionable technologies and procedures. The Institute of Medicine defines technology assessment as the "process of examining and reporting properties of medical technology used in health care, such as safety, efficacy, feasibility and indications for use, cost, and cost-effectiveness, as well as social, economic, and ethical considerations, whether intended or unintended." This definition alludes to two aspects of HTA that are critical for its full effectiveness: a concern with the broad effects on society and a more subtle emphasis on second-order consequences, which are unintended, indirect, or delayed. Any assessment of health technologies or the proposed programs to be built around them must focus on both of these concerns as well as on the strictly technical questions of safety and efficacy, which often receive predominant attention.

In 1982, the Office of Technology Assessment (OTA)

described the context of HTA at that time as one where "Federal agencies and private insurers and organizations set policies, guidelines, regulations, and/or make reimbursement coverage determinations, many of which profoundly affect the adoption and level of use of medical technologies. Yet, their decisions are usually based on informal, subjective, group-generated norms which tend to support the status quo." Unfortunately, its observations remain relevant today. No class of medical technology is adequately evaluated on a continuing basis for either cost effectiveness or social or ethical implications. Despite widespread efforts at HTA, there is no single organization whose mission it is to ensure that medical and surgical procedures are fully assessed before their widespread use. The result is a loosely structured, largely private collection of efforts lacking centralized guidance or control. As David Banta described it in 2003:

> No class of medical technology is adequately evaluated on a continuing basis for either cost effectiveness or social or ethical implications. Despite widespread efforts at Health Technology Assessment (HTA), there is no single organization whose mission it is to assure that medical and surgical procedures are fully assessed before their widespread use.

> The overall impact of HTA in the United States is impossible to evaluate. With no effective national co-ordination, HTA activities are carried out in many organizations with different goals in mind, often using different methods. The predominant goal is probably cost-containment, but other goals, such as improving quality or innovation, are also strongly supported by some powerful actors in the system. In short, however, the United States has no coherent policy concerning either health technology or HTA.

Furthermore, the synthesis phase of HTA continues to be weak at best. As evidenced by the recent expansion of coverage for heart and liver transplantations and funding of AIDS research and treatment, reimbursement and regulatory decisions continue to be under the heavy influence of the political climate and clearly reflect a value system mired in the technological imperative.

It is understandable that HTA has had opposition from many forces within the medical industry. Because such assessment takes time, it threatens to delay new technology applications and thus dampen potential profits. Any attempts to stop or slow development of particular medical innovations, therefore, face strong criticism from those who have a stake in continued funding. Ironically, this opposition, in part, has been a factor in shaping HTA efforts such that they are largely ineffective in controlling the proliferation of medical innovations. In turn, this has raised a competing set of criticisms from those who feel that HTA is bound to fail because it does not challenge assumptions of the medical model and the technological imperative.

According to Daniel Callahan, the HTA movement is just another example of the faith-in-technology fixes for complex social problems because it lacks any real value framework by which to make judgments on the moral or social worth or value of different technological goals. It can assess relative efficacy and economic consequences, but it cannot help determine the justice of bearing these consequences. Janine Morgall, too, contends that HTA has not moved beyond the status quo and is built upon the assumptions of the medical model. As a result, "the possibility of totally rejecting the technology in question is not really an option in most methods, which do not challenge the technology but rather take it as given." To do otherwise, of course, would go not only against the interests of the medical industry, but also against the strong predisposition among the American public to support development of technologies that might benefit individuals, no matter how costly.

The result of these value preferences is an almost universal failure of HTA to recommend against development of even highly questionable techniques or to reassess older technologies and consider discontinuing their use. Part of this problem might stem from an inherent difficulty of HTA to deal with futuristic problems. Whether because of short-term political pressures, the difficulty of forecasting long-term problems, or some combination of both, the time frame of HTA continues to be limited to the near future. Moreover, the strong preference of the public and leaders for quick diffusion of advanced biomedical interventions makes any attempts to restrict their development politically unattractive. The burden these technologies may place on future generations by intensifying hope and expectations and the negative consequences that might accompany them are thus minimized or even absent from most assessments.

> The strong preference of the public and leaders for quick diffusion of advanced biomedical interventions makes any attempts to restrict their development politically unattractive.

Because HTA lacks the capacity to critically analyze the prevailing value framework itself, it is an inadequate tool for making hard choices. A common assumption of HTA is that if a technology is safe and effective, it should be used and funded. America cannot blindly continue such a shallow standard. Because, as Callahan notes, efficacy and affordability are two entirely different matters, and their implicit conflation in such technology assessment promotion contributes enormously to the illusion that the key to cost containment lies in determining which technologies will be efficacious. This could well be called the *efficacy fallacy*: if it works, we should therefore be able to afford it.

As unlikely as it is for HTA to reject a technology because it is ineffective or futile, it is even less likely that efficacious and safe technologies, but unaffordable ones, will be rejected. As argued earlier, however, elimination of ineffective technologies alone will not resolve the health care crisis. Hard decisions involve sacrificing clinically useful technologies, technologies that may work but that collectively might bankrupt the system while contributing very little to the health of the population. There must be a willingness to engage in prospective assessment before technologies are introduced and to force a discontinuation of the use of those technologies that are ineffective or only marginally effective, or effective but too expensive to find social justification.

Another criticism leveled indirectly at HTA is that though it might free up resources by improving, at least marginally, the precision of medical care, an unstated assumption is that the resources saved will be redeployed elsewhere in medical care, not shifted to nonmedical health initiatives that might be more effective. Jonathan Lomas and Andre-Pierre Contandriopoulos state it succinctly in saying, "The redirection of such resources to alternative [nonmedical] pathways to better population health is not contemplated, and in the absence of coordination with the public, regulation will not occur."

Although at its best, HTA can tell us whether we are doing things right within the context of medical care, it cannot tell us whether we are doing the right things for the maintenance and promotion of the health of the population, because by focusing only on the former, we leave out nonmedical possibilities for improving health.

Despite the increasing magnitude and frequency of HTA, most efforts continue to be flawed. Furthermore, the failure of such assessments has less to do with the capabilities of the assessing agents or even the strategies and methods used than it does with the value context underlying medicine. The constraints, then, are political and social and reflect the high personal stakes that are inherent in the life and death issues surrounding health policy. The failure of all but a small minority of HTA efforts to flatly reject certain directions of research or even to place a low priority on them is not surprising given the potentially explosive nature of such recommendations. Moreover, in those few cases where such recommendations have been made (for example, with the artificial heart), the political response has been predictable and the HTA has been ignored.

> The failure of all but a small minority of HTA efforts to flatly reject certain directions of research or even to place a low priority on them is not surprising given the potentially explosive nature of such recommendations.

A reevaluation of these values that now constrain HTA is urgently needed. Again, this is not a new idea. The 1976 OTA report concluded that macro-alternatives to each technology being assessed should be defined, alternative strategies to solve the same medical problem in different ways be explored, and the effect that the technology in question will have on the development and implementation of those alternatives be considered.

"For example, in assessing a therapeutic technology, one might consider proposals for prevention of the disease in question. It would be legitimate, in this context, to ask how reasonable, feasible, or desirable these alternatives are and whether heavy investment in or implementation of the therapeutic technology would encourage, discourage, or complement their development and implementation." Due to the process by which candidates are selected for assessment, and the often narrowly focused requests that limit the scope of a particular study, discussion of macro-alternatives, particularly nontechnological ones, is frequently limited or absent in HTA final reports. The strong value bias in favor of technological fixes for individual patients combined with the inherent dramatic nature of many interventions creates a strong resistance against either rejecting the technological solutions or recommending alternative nontechnological strategies.

Health Outcomes Impact Statements

The inability of HTA to constrain the medical model should be no surprise in light of the model's cherished place in the American value system. Despite the best intentions and efforts of the assessors, it is virtually impossible to break out of the confines created by society. Under conventional HTA, the process places the burden of proof on those people or groups who would block new technologies and procedures, a virtually impossible task given the vagaries and complexities of medical science. Any reasonable doubts are resolved in favor of going ahead with development, diffusion, and eventually funding of the technology in question. If we are serious about assuring that medical innovations (and existing practices) are indeed safe, effective, and efficient in producing health, the burden of proof for demonstration must be shifted to the innovations' proponents. This would put medical procedures on more equal grounds with drugs and biologics. Callahan is correct when he concludes that in weighing the consequences of technologies, we should assume the worst outcome and put the burden on the optimists to prove the assumption wrong: "We have reached a point in medical progress where we can begin to assume that, unless proved otherwise, the consequences of medical advances are as likely to be harmful as beneficial—and that is precisely because we have made so much progress already, making future progress not less likely, but more problematical in its beneficial outcome."

> In weighing the consequences of technologies, we should assume the worst outcome and put the burden on the optimists to prove the assumption wrong.

To this end, we should institute the concept of a health outcomes impact statement analogous to environmental impact statements. Under such an approach, the purveyors of new technologies or particularly new intervention areas such as neural grafting and preimplantation genetics would by law need to attain approval from a health outcomes board before they could claim status as a clinical procedure and receive public health care dollars. Without such approval, the intervention would remain on a preclinical or experimental status. More importantly, the burden of proof not only for safety and efficacy, but also as to its contribution to health would be rigorous, thus denying approval to intervention areas that were judged insufficient by these criteria. Although the health outcomes board would not have the authority to prohibit use of any techniques or procedures, reimbursement through the public health care budget could not occur prior to preliminary approval, nor would private insurers be under any obligation to reimburse them. Furthermore, any patients who underwent the intervention would have to be informed of its status regarding health outcomes.

Although this proposal is bound to be attacked as unduly slowing medical progress and as unjustified interference with medical prerogative, it is not a revolutionary concept. Other countries in effect do this on a regular basis through a variety of mechanisms such as the National Institute for Clinical Excellence in the United Kingdom, the Investigational Medicine Fund in the Netherlands, and the Swedish Council for Technology Assessment in Health Care in Sweden. Before new techniques or procedures are reimbursed, proponents must demonstrate that the innovation will do the job better than existing methods and/or do it in a more cost-effective way. Obviously, such an approach is considerably more difficult in a private-oriented health system with no global budgets, though Japan has managed to do this with their national fee structure. However, given the current crises in health benefits, employers and private insurers should embrace a process that protects them from paying for unproven and unapproved techniques. The proposed health outcomes impact approach would go a step further by requiring evidence of a clear contribution to population health in proportion to the cost of the innovation, thus addressing the concern that alternative, nonmedical pathways to health be considered on an equal basis when assessing medical technologies.

Need for Anticipatory Policy

Whatever approach is taken, whether to broaden technology assessments or institute health outcomes impact statements, there is an urgent need for anticipatory policy founded in transparent goals as to where we want to be in ten years, twenty years, and beyond. What type of society do we want to leave our children, and where does health fit into this? We have allowed to flourish an uncontrolled health care arena that has set unrealistic precedents that cannot be sustained—we cannot continue relying on ad hoc, reactive policy making any longer. The question no longer is whether to set societal limits; the questions are how and by whom.

What agency can make anticipatory policy? Unlike other Western nations, to date the U.S. government has not intervened directly to set limits, instead trying to encourage demand-side constraints for cost containment and assuming that providers, insurers, and the public will somehow muddle through. Without strict policy guidance, however, the medical profession has avoided sharing responsibility for resource allocation activities while the insured public is skeptical of reforms that threaten to encroach on their preferences and benefits. At the broadest level, the debate in the United States has centered on a dichotomy between public and private regulation of medical care. Although the public has ultimate responsibility for the health of the population, the dominance of the medical model and the power of the private sector mean that the predominant proportion of health care has remained the domain of nonpublic interests, even as the share paid by the public has escalated.

Traditionally in the United States, the practice of medicine, as distinguished from public health, has been treated as a private matter between the health professional and the patient. Although professional ethics and standards of practice provided a guide to clinician discretion, overall the individual physician held considerable autonomy. The emergence of professional societies and the increased nationalization of standards shifted professional control from individual practitioners to state and national organizations, but nevertheless were acceptable to most clinicians for the protections they offered to those who adhered to their professional guidelines. This shift was also viewed as preventing more active government involvement. By presenting itself as a profession, medicine has deflected public examination of the health professional–patient relationship. Although the self-regulation approach has largely served the medical community and individual patients well, it has discouraged resource allocation efforts and reinforced the dominance of the medical model to the exclusion of society-wide considerations. It has meant that "decisions to use sophisticated and sometimes invasive [and expensive] medical technologies are being made almost solely by those who have been trained to use that technology," as noted by Benjamin Fuller.

There is, however, a paradox in arguing for more public involvement in health policy. Given the American value system and the strong belief of the public in the illusions of medicine, heightened public involvement might solidify support for the dominant medical model. If the value system as we have described it is accurate, it is unlikely that more attention to the public will do much to resolve the problems. In fact, if the public really demanded the needed changes, policy shifts in that direction would have already been forthcoming. What is needed, then, is not simply a broadened debate, but an enlightened one led by courageous leaders who are willing to fight for the necessary conceptual and practical changes. Health care reform appears to be one area where the value system effectively works against change that is critical to the public's health, both literally and figuratively.

It may very well be that the only way to make the hard decisions necessary to reform the health care system in the fragmented and incremental American system would be to adopt the strategy offered by Paul Light. In his book on the Bipartisan Commission on Social Security, Light concludes that there are certain public issues that are best dealt with in secret negotiations outside of the public spotlight. Those issues that involve cutting benefits or raising taxes, rather than distributing the government largess, he terms "de-distributive." Health care issues appear to be a prime example of such issues that can never be resolved in the public forum because they elicit insurmountable opposition from powerful interests on many sides. According to Light, with the public and interest groups firmly opposed to most of the major options in the de-distributive agenda, Congress and the president are well advised to build prenegotiated packages outside the constitutional system, returning to the normal process only at the last minute. In light of the continuing paralysis of traditional U.S. political institutions to make the necessary changes to the U.S. health care system, strategies of the type described by Light ought to be given serious consideration. The mandate given such a multipartisan body should focus on defining the broader goals of medicine and making suggestions as to how best to achieve these goals within the context described here. Whatever is done, however, should be done now rather than delayed until the health care meltdown occurs.

Chapter 5
Where Do We Go from Here?

The future of health care is inextricably tied to the future of America as a self-governing entity. This is not just another issue: we must control health care spending (and correct the injustice of leaving over 40 million people uninsured) or we will undercut our economy and America's position in the world. America is now spending four times the percentage of its GDP on health care as we do on defense, and that cost is rising at over twice the rate of inflation. It is America's fiscal black hole, and, at the same time, the biggest failure in our social contract.

The stakes involved go even further. The question of health care and entitlements generally go to the heart of America's ability to sustain a democracy. A new issue has arisen that we have never heretofore had to consider: Is our political system structured to be able to solve the problems the nation faces? Can we do politically what we must do economically and socially to leave our children a workable and decent society? Before you discard these questions as heresy, remember that many of our most famous Greek philosophers felt that democracy was not a sustainable form of government. No less an American as founding father John Adams warned that democracy "wastes, exhausts, and murders itself. There was never a democracy yet that did not commit suicide."

Can we ever stop the slide toward national insolvency, which will collapse the dollar and undercut the economy? Even though different studies produce different figures, most of the experts and organizations that worry about the national budget agree that we are passing on to our children debts higher than the total worth of the public and private wealth of the country. The Concord Coalition puts the national debt plus the unfunded liabilities at over $70 trillion, substantially more than the nation's total public and private assets. We are clearly the most fiscally irresponsible generation in American history, and neither political party can take even modest steps to balance the budget.

Every dime of the war in Iraq, the recovery from Hurricane Katrina, every dime of the new avian flu program and a thousand other federal programs we callously sloughed off to our children and grandchildren to pay. Some of these programs may indeed be worthy, but when we cut taxes without cutting spending, we do not cut taxes but instead pass the burden along to our children. We have made promises far beyond our ability to deliver and left the political consequences to our children.

Some would contend that this is much too dark a view of America's future. We understand that America has been a brilliant problem-solving machine. But generally, American history has been one of distributing the spoils of a rich continent. Seldom, outside of war, has America called on its citizens for sacrifice. Yet that is what must happen. One basic problem we refuse to recognize is that the New Deal is demographically obsolete. Medicare, Medicaid, and Social Security are the most politically popular programs in America, but none of them are sustainable without major political career–destroying amendments. We are living too long and not having enough children to sustain these programs, yet we are paralyzed to act. By 2030, there will be twice as many elderly and only 18 percent more children, and these three programs alone will crowd out all the rest of federal spending.

The programs bankrupting America are programs for the elderly paid for by today's workers. These programs slowly but steadily put new, impossible burdens on these workers' children, our children, and everybody's grandchildren. Consequently, day by day, decision by decision, budget by budget, we consign our nation's children

> Our generation, however, for the first time, is leaving gargantuan unresolved problems to the future. But our worst nightmare is that these problems might be beyond the ability of democracy to solve.

and grandchildren to economic chaos. We are and will increasingly see workers paying over 15 percent of their wages into programs that benefit seniors who on average make more in retirement that they did working full time. In addition, health care costs represent one of the fastest growing items in both business and family budgets.

It is no great feat to sustain a democracy when we are distributing the riches of a virgin, resource-rich continent. With notable exceptions during world wars and the Depression, our political system gave voters more and more benefits every decade. When we could not pay for those benefits, we started to put them on our children's credit card. It is no big deal if we add debt temporarily for a short-term crisis, but debt is "economic cocaine," and we have become addicted to debt. We are haunted by the fact that every generation of Americans until ours has left its children a better America. Our generation, however, for the first time, is leaving gargantuan unresolved problems to the future. But our worst nightmare is that these problems might be beyond the ability of democracy to solve.

The former president of France M. Valéry Giscard d'Estaing once observed that "Politics is not the art of the possible. It is the art of making what is necessary possible." Wise words, and most appropriate to the health care dilemma. If democracy is to work and sustain itself, it must successfully face and solve the major issues it is confronted with and do so in a timely manner. In contrast, we are currently deferring, not solving, the major issues confronting America, and our inaction is becoming nation threatening. Nothing less than the future of our country is at stake.

The former president of France M. Valéry Giscard d'Estaing once observed that "Politics is not the art of the possible. It is the art of making what is necessary possible." Wise words, and most appropriate to the health care dilemma.

Being in government and having to balance a budget is like sleeping with a blanket that is too small. You pull the blanket up around your shoulders and your feet get cold. You cover your feet and your chest gets cold. There is never enough of the blanket to cover all the needs. This is a hard reality for Americans to learn. Governing requires making choices and funding them, not deferring them to future generations. Ultimately any nation cannot create social justice on borrowed money. It will merely create injustice for our kids and grandkids. At the core of this growing national tragedy is health care.

The Crisis in Health Care

The task facing U.S. society in reordering the health system is Herculean in scope and requires a reevaluation of the basic values and beliefs of all Americans. It also necessitates a reassessment of the purpose of government and what type of society we want to be. The crisis in the health system, like the emerging crisis in Social Security and the continuing problems of immigration and racial equality, go

> We no longer have the luxury of constructing our health care system an individual at a time. We need a wider vision of health in society and of how we keep our society healthy.

to the core of our view of what we are. By relying on incremental, nonplanned policy to guide us, we have given up the capacity to exert effective control over the forces of technology. This failure to appreciate long-term implications of our policies is nowhere more evident than in our skewed health priorities and our dependence on the medical model to provide health.

To bring health care spending under control, we must rethink its very basic assumptions. We must not only rebuild our health care system, but (first) we must rebuild our thinking about the structure of duties and responsibilities in health care. We no longer have the luxury of constructing our health care system an individual at a time. We need a wider vision of health in society and of how we keep our society healthy. In the words of William Kraus:

> As more and more of our national wealth is being allocated to sophisticated medical services like intensive care, it becomes more and more likely that the extraordinary demands of a few desperately ill individuals or the indiscriminate application of a new expensive treatment will threaten the availability of basic medical services.

As we have demonstrated in earlier chapters, this state of affairs is not only patently unfair, but also unsustainable.

Calling U.S. health care a "system" in itself stretches any imaginable use of that term, which implies order and some underlying logic. In effect, health care in the United States has evolved without either order or logic, much like a flight when air traffic control is on holiday, with no clear destination, and with pilots in disagreement as to what to do and where to go. Further, flight attendants are competing for passenger attention while complaining of pay cuts and limits imposed on them. Meanwhile, while first-class passengers are enjoying the best of services, many economy-class passengers are demanding first-class services while complaining about the costs of the flight, and those in the back of the plane get no pretzels because those up front got them all. No one in their right mind would sign on for such a flight, but Americans as a whole accept this disarray in health care and reject calls for methodical control of health care as undesirable and against their best interests.

> Health care in the United States has evolved without either order or logic, much like a flight when air traffic control is on holiday, with no clear destination, and with pilots in disagreement as to what to do and where to go.

This lack of control of health care is exacerbated by an aging population, the continued development and diffusion of new medical technologies, and heightened public expectations. Unless major changes are made soon, chaos will emerge. Because we can do little if anything to affect the aging population, our options are largely restricted to altering medical technology diffusion and public demands and expectations. Taking control of our destiny by constraining medical technology and lowering public expectations for it, however, conflicts directly with the contemporary economic incentive structure, our individual-oriented value system, and our faith in a medical model driven by an ever-expanding array of technologies. Society has to decide whether to continue to shift resources from other social areas and from future generations to satisfy our insatiable appetite for health care.

Any moves toward restructuring the health care system must be accompanied by widespread public education on the limits of medicine and the need to set difficult priorities so as to get the most out of our investment in health care. Because the technological imperative is sustained as much by public demand as by corporate and professional control, efforts must be made to reduce public demand for medical services. This can be accomplished only by placing more emphasis on individual responsibility for health and on health promotion, disease prevention, and environmental health.

The dismal record of funding for health education as a proportion of total health care expenditures must be remedied. Most important is the need to instill in the public the value of collective self-restraint. At present, neither patients nor providers are conditioned toward this end. The current structure of third-party reimbursement (either public or private) without external constraints provides a compelling predisposition to consume extensive resources, because individual patients bear at best a small proportion of the costs for the benefits they accrue. The incentive is always to use more—to demand that all be done that technically can be done—especially near the end of life.

As discussed in Chapter 2, a moral hazard arises when consumers of health care assess medical needs without considering the full price. Because needs largely define demand, there is an inherent bias in the system toward intensified demand. However, as stated by Ruth

Chadwick, if "we allow individuals or groups to define their own needs, we will be subject to the bottomless pit problem." Although a large proportion of the American public agrees that cost containment in health care is essential, few are willing to sacrifice currently held benefits in order to reduce overall costs to society, nor are they motivated to make drastic lifestyle changes or stay physically fit out of a responsibility to reduce the overall cost of health care. By focusing on the individual at the cost of the collectivity, America has painted itself into a corner from which escape will be difficult, indeed painful. However, the longer we delay in facing the reality of limits and making necessary changes, the more problematic the task and the fewer the options.

> The longer we delay in facing the reality of limits and making necessary changes, the more problematic the task and the fewer the options.

Although the themes discussed in this book have provoked debate within the academic community and in some state legislatures, overall there has been little discussion in any national forum. Instead of confronting these more basic questions regarding the goals of health care and challenging misconceptions regarding needed constraints, talk of reform has been directed toward expanding existing levels of health care coverage, shifting even more resources to the elderly, and containing costs painlessly through better management. The forces against major change from the status quo are imposing and include politicians who are afraid to say no, a powerful health care industry with high stakes in ever more spending, a medical profession heavily skewed toward specialists, a legal system that encourages defensive medicine, and a public that expects the best of care paid, of course, by a third party. All the institutions and the workforce in health care are structured for more and more spending. There are no effective restraints. It is all sail and no anchor. Not surprisingly, recognizing the need to ration medical resources, the advantages of adopting an expanded model of health, the necessity of setting some form of equitable global limits, and the need to ensure the collective health of society remains largely absent.

The Levels of Health Care and Moral Duty

As introduced in Chapter 1, part of the problem we face in the United States is the failure to recognize or at least admit that there are different levels of moral responsibility in health care similar to different levels of a building. The first floor is the ethics and duties of the doctor-patient relationship and individual responsibility. The foundation of the house of health care is self-responsibility. No nation can ignore the causes of poor health and only deal with the consequences. That includes new obligations on individuals to avoid harmful lifestyles. Although taxing cigarettes and alcohol is relatively easy, the task of setting new responsibilities on people for their own health is difficult, but necessary. This requires challenging the prevailing orthodoxies of patient and physician autonomy. Americans' sense of autonomy, which seems to mean that all Americans have a right to unlimited high-technology medicine, is obsolete and has to be challenged. We can give people almost unlimited care, but not unlimited cure, especially when they refuse to behave in ways that maximize their health.

Other countries, especially those with national health

services, such as Great Britain, put considerable emphasis on the role of the individual and deny costly services to those who fail to make lifestyle changes. This is easier to do with a global budget because it is clear that resources used on one self-destructive individual could be better allocated to others in the system. In the United States, however, in the absence of explicit trade-offs, priorities, or centralized responsibility, such a policy is viewed by many as punishment, as blaming the victim. This is most unfortunate, because punishment is not the objective, but rather some sense of equity and fairness. The reality is that resources are limited and that the "opportunity costs" of money spent on self-abusive diseases can buy much more health in other places in the system. We should be compassionately allocating with a broader moral vision, which is not the same as punishing. We simply can't allow people to endlessly abuse their bodies and then expect society to underwrite their cure. As noted by Tristram Engelhardt, "There are moral as well as financial limits to society's protection of its members from the risk of poor health." Even more so where that poor health is self-imposed.

> We should be compassionately allocating with a broader moral vision, which is not the same as punishing.

Even in cases where the person has not contributed to her or his own ill health, there must be new limits and new realization on the part of Americans that those limits are necessary, proper, and just. No one has a right to unlimited care. A major problem over rights in the United States is the failure to distinguish between negative and positive rights. Negative rights relate to the freedom to be left alone to use one's resources as one sees fit, whereby the only claim on others is a freedom from intrusion.

Health care as a negative right would allow patients with adequate personal resources to use them to maximize their use of health care. In contrast, positive rights impose obligations on others (society) to provide those goods and services necessary for each individual to exercise her or his rights. This more expansive notion of rights requires the presence of institutions that guarantee a certain level of material well-being, through governmental redistribution of resources, where necessary. Although in liberal U.S. society it would be nearly impossible to impose limits on the negative rights of individuals to use whatever medicine they can afford, there must be limits on what individuals can claim as positive rights. Even though all citizens have a positive right to basic health services, limits can justifiably be set on entitlements to health care. Although a person has a right to say no in the health care system (for example, to discontinue a life support system), this does not extend to a positive right to endlessly tap public funds for care.

The second floor of health care is made up of the ethics and duties of the community and health insurance plans, whose financial and moral obligation is to the total group whose premiums make up the money under their control. The third floor of health care is the state and nation. Neither the second nor the third floor of health care can give the Hippocratic oath a blank check. As cogently offered by a Chinese proverb, "The normal physician treats the problem. The good physician treats the person. The best physician treats the community." Our current doctrines of personal autonomy and professional autonomy are unsustainable. They are nation-bankrupting doctrines in a time of high-technology medicine. Technology in its expensive creativity has undercut autonomy. As Victor

Fuchs argues, "The divergence between what is good for the patient and what is efficient for society as a whole is a key element in current concerns over health care spending." Moreover, Fuch's concept of "substituted mortality and substituted morbidity" becomes important here. When you are funding a health plan, no one is ever "cured," but rather they are temporarily fixed so they can get sick later of something else. Thus, the decision to treat at one point often leads to a series of increasingly difficult decisions as to where to draw the line, much like with an aging car that becomes a money pit with one major investment followed by another. Although this fact in itself should not negate initial treatment, it must be a major consideration on the third floor of health care.

We need new ethical analyses to determine the role of the health plan and government and to better evaluate their fiduciary duty in the funding of health care. All three levels of analysis are necessarily related but not coterminous. Only when the American public understands that rationing is unavoidable on the top two floors can we begin to truly revamp our health care system. As stated by Daniel Callahan, "We will not be able to work out the problems of our health care system unless we shift our priorities and bias from an individual-centered to a community-centered view of health and human welfare." Every community and every health plan grapples with limited resources and has to think about how to optimize health with limited funds. For those who doubt this, Ernie Young concludes that "Limits must be considered if costs are to be held down and universal access to the system is to be guaranteed. Quality can and must be maintained but not quantity. Marginally beneficial or useless treatments are inimical to quality medical care."

Once we start to think of the moral radius of the second and third floor of health care, we see that there is a conflict in utilitarianism; we cannot provide the greatest good to the greatest number. The greatest good is at war with the greatest number. There is an inevitable trade-off. Physician and patient autonomy under the assumption of unlimited resources must give way to a system where the health plan has a duty to maximize health within available resources. Then the focus changes from the individual patient to the entire membership of the plan. As stated by Haavi Morreim in discussing her concept of contributive justice, "All members of the group give up a small benefit, but receive in return a larger benefit, i.e., the ability of the group to optimize the dollars available." She points out that to give a particular patient everything he and his doctor wants is unethical because "generous compassion for one is inevitably bought at the expense of the many whose contributions create and who in turn rely on the common resource pool." The second floor has a responsibility to its entire membership, and this inevitably means having to say yes in one place and no in another. Rationing of resources is, therefore, unavoidable on both the second and third floors. The membership can demand that it be fair and that it be transparent, but they cannot demand that it not exist. It is inherent in their role. All who distribute limited funds have to live forever forward under what Morreim termed "conditions of fiscal scarcity."

The third floor of health care is the state or nation. It is here that a new prominence must be placed. At this level, the greatest impact can be achieved. There are two threshold questions for the state or nation: "Who?" and "How?" "Who" relates to who will be covered. All citizens and all others legally in the country should be covered. In contrast, it would be unfair for a person to get a visa or come into the country illegally for delivery of a child, fertility treatment, or cancer treatment at public expense. What, if any, duty do we owe tourists? If noncitizens are here legally and are working and paying taxes, they should be covered by the state or nation to the same extent as citizens, but if they are not, they should be denied community funds.

The most important question on the third floor is "How do we keep the nation healthy?" The ancient Greeks used to say, "To know all to ask is to know half." This aphorism is important to health policy. Once we ask how we keep the nation healthy, the dilemma is half solved. A nation's health is much broader than its health care system, and policy makers must lift their eyes from only recognizing the individual patient. Policy makers have many options other than health care to produce health in a society. As Fuchs notes, "Income, education, occupation, age, sex, marital status, and ethnicity are all correlated with health in one context or another. ... Effective health policy requires an understanding of these correlations."

There is substantial evidence that health status is highly correlated with socioeconomic status. If a primary goal of health policy is to improve the health status of the population, it is crucial to focus on economic and social determinants of health. This requires a shift away from the dominance of the medical care system toward this more inclusive model of health. Lower social class as measured by income, education, or other socioeconomic status indicators is related with higher death rates overall and higher rates of most diseases that are the most common causes of death. The best health results are achieved in those societies that minimize the gap between the rich and the poor. At a cross-national level, research consistently shows that the health of the population has more to do with the distribution of income than it does with the level of medical spending. Importantly, social class differences in mortality and morbidity continue to widen as the income divide between rich and poor widens.

Even though there is little doubt that medical care can be decisive in individual cases, there is substantial evidence to demonstrate that it is but a minor determinant of the health of a population. If the goal of health care is to improve the health of the population as a whole, then the medical model must be reassessed.

> The best health results are achieved in those societies that minimize the gap between the rich and the poor.

Three decades ago, Ivan Illich vehemently criticized modern medicine as a nemesis and a cause, not a cure, of illness. Although Illich's criticisms of medicine were unduly harsh, he raised many legitimate questions. There is strong support, for instance, for his conclusion that major improvements in health derive from changes in the way in which people are able to live, not medical intervention. Too much medicine is not good for health. Not only does it divert resources from more useful endeavors, but it also can actually produce ill health, as demonstrated by the large number of deaths attributed to treatment each year in the United States. Furthermore, medicine can disrupt traditional social and cultural institutions and values that are central to good health in the broader sense, even notions of the natural death, as Laurine Graig details:

An explosion in medical knowledge and technology has allowed us to redefine our relationship with death. Our belief in science has limited our acceptance of death as divine or natural providence. ... Theoretically, one could now spend all of his or her available time and money in the pursuit of health.

The focus on medical care is also flawed because it elevates health as a primary goal instead of a means to broader life goals. Health must be put into perspective along with a wide array of elements of an enjoyable life, including art, entertainment, music, work, as well as family and social interaction. To place health above everything else risks underestimating the contribution of these many other factors to the fulfillment of our goals and the enhancement of the human condition. We cannot live by health alone but must invest in education, infrastructure, and other essential components. Although health is important, it is not all-important. It makes little sense to invest disproportionate amounts of societal resources into health at the sacrifice of those things that make life worth living. Unfortunately, Americans expect the health care system to resolve many problems that at their core are not medical ones.

> The focus on medical care is also flawed because it elevates health as a primary goal instead of a means to broader life goals.

Implicit in the conventional health care model is the assumption that improved health status is achieved primarily by higher expenditures on medical care. Although the health status of individuals is influenced by medical care and it has the potential to improve quality of life or extend the lives of some people, there is little correlation between how much money is spent on doctors and hospitals and the health of society. As noted earlier, though the United States spends considerably more than other countries on medical care, it is far down the list on health outcomes on most measures. The impact of medical care is further limited because many health conditions are self-limiting, some are incurable, and for many others, there is little or no effective treatment. As Fuchs remarks, the cases where health care is effective and significantly affects health outcomes "comprise only a small proportion of total medical care—too small to make a discernible impact on the statistics in populations."

> If we are serious about maximizing the health of the population, resources are best directed toward alleviating poverty, reducing crime and violence, and changing lifestyles.

These findings regarding the inadequacy of explaining health status by health care have significant implications for any efforts to restructure the health care system. If we are serious about maximizing the health of the population, resources are best directed toward alleviating poverty, reducing crime and violence, and changing lifestyles. A healthy person does not need medical care. Our goal should be to keep people and thus the population as healthy as possible.

Rationing health care requires politics based on judgments about fairness. With this in mind, we should view each state legislature as a giant ethics committee. Moreover, federal legislators have a coterminous moral responsibility to institute a workable, just rationing scheme and make the difficult decisions outlined here. The uninsured lie within government's moral radius. The abrogation of this responsibility by all but a few of the states and by the federal government is a black mark on all political parties. Most difficult to accept are decisions such as that by

Jeb Bush as governor of Florida in the Terri Schiavo case, which demonstrated a clear lack of moral insight at this level. At the time he was taking all possible legal action to extend care for one person in a persistent vegetative state against the wishes of her husband, Florida had 2.9 million uninsured people (the percentage of Florida's residents uninsured at the time was over 21 percent, as opposed to a national average of 17 percent). A governor and state legislature must survey the entire battlefield when making their judgments. Legislators should be judged not only for what they do, but also for what they do not do. We must start to make them aware of the full moral scope of their position and demand that they explain such actions in light of their broader responsibility to the public.

Every governing body should broadly examine how it can bring health to its constituents. Governments can avoid the issue, as most do now in the United States, but they cannot evade the moral responsibility we put on them.

Medical ethics' major emphasis on the individual results in unethical public policy. It looks too narrowly and with one eye. At the state or national level we must get beyond the patient view and think about the implications to the broader society. Rene Fox views medical ethics in just this narrow way: "Bioethics deals ... with nothing less than beliefs, values and norms that are basic to our society, its cultural tradition, and its collective conscience." This is not only myopic, but also harmful. Frank Lewins expands further on this idea:

> Much of the literature on bioethics is narrow because it overlooks the social context in which ethical decisions and ethical dilemmas occur. Consequently, the impression running through that literature is that bioethical issues

are best understood and resolved by examining the nature of bioethics rather than the situation in which bioethical issues arise.

Now that government pays approximately 60 percent of U.S. health care, more than ever we must look at these issues in a broader social context.

Responsibility to Future Generations

Another conspicuous absence from the contemporary debate over health care reform is the impact of our actions on future generations. Although some observers explicitly call for restraint by the current generation out of concern for our children and others make reference to how we will retire the baby boomers, by and large we treat the issue of health reform solely in terms of the needs of those now living. Our overspending today, however, markedly affects future generations, first by creating an imponderable national debt and second by setting unrealistic precedents and expectations that can be upheld only at great expense to a shrinking younger population.

> Collective health of society must be broadened to take into account the impact of our goals and priorities on those who follow.

The shift in emphasis from individual health to collective health in itself, then, is not enough. Collective health of society must be broadened to take into account the impact of our goals and priorities on those who follow. This challenges the very foundations of liberal Western ethics, which presupposes that the sphere of human action does not reach beyond the present and immediate. Under prevailing ethical frameworks, the time span of goal setting and accountability is short, and

proper conduct is defined by immediate or near consequences only. In the wake of endless and costly modern
technologies, however, all of this has drastically and
irreparably changed. With the newfound powers we have
to reshape nature and alter the human condition come
the corresponding ethical responsibility for the exercise
of these powers. Simply put, we must enlarge the concept of justice to include intergenerational equity. Under
this ethics of responsibility, an agent's concrete moral
responsibility at the time of action extends far beyond its
proximate effects.

The integration of a proper concern for the future
into the policy-making process necessitates substantial
alterations in the way we as a society make decisions. In
fact, this new responsibility casts doubt on the capacity
of representative government, as now practiced, to meet
these demands. Under a pluralist system, only present
interests make themselves heard and felt and require
consideration by policy makers. Especially on issues as
complex and emotionally charged as setting priorities for
health care, single-issue interest groups become active,
vocal, and influential. With few exceptions, their concern is with the near-term or immediate, not the distant
future. Also, because public officials are held accountable
to their constituencies of the present, future-oriented
policy is sacrificed to placating those people and groups
whose demands are loudest. The future, however important, too often is trumped by the immediate. Because
the interests of the day hold sway, the future is nowhere
represented. The seemingly imminent is always at war
with the truly important.

Moreover, the current election system, with its
dependence on political action committee contributions,

clearly exacerbates the inability and unwillingness to look beyond the next election. As long as policy makers are reelected on the basis of what they do for present-oriented interests, there remains a strong disincentive to become actively embroiled in controversial issues of the future. It is easier to avoid these "no-win" issues and ignore or obscure the long-term consequences of public

> As long as policy makers are reelected on the basis of what they do for present-oriented interests, there remains a strong disincentive to become actively embroiled in controversial issues of the future.

inaction than recognize the ethics of responsibility to the future. Workable strategies to overcome this impasse and ensure proper consideration of these policy problems, then, require consideration of creative, even revolutionary, innovations in assessment mechanisms.

What to Do? Needed Changes

The resolution of the health care crisis will require making harder choices than the U.S. population and its representatives have to date been willing to consider. The following changes are essential if we are to have any chance of meeting the goal of collective health in the coming decades.

First, we must institute a system of universal coverage for a set of basic services with copayments based on income. That we are the only industrialized country without some form of guaranteed health care is a crime.

Second, we must move toward a transparent, explicit rationing system for care above this basic package for costly medical care. This will require inclusion of clear cost-benefit criteria and preclude the prevailing weight placed on unlimited and often inappropriate treatment regimes. Although setting categorical limits and a prioritized or core-services format to rationing services is necessary, there is an array of explicit non-price, supply-side rationing strategies that could be considered. The main point, however, is to establish as fair and equitable an approach to setting limits as possible. We must realize, however, that any rationing system will mean denial of potentially beneficial services to certain identifiable patients.

Third, we need to clarify the relationship between individual behavior and ill health. Despite dangers of victim blaming, we have to assign individual responsibility for ill health that is clearly related to deleterious behavior. Although all people should have access to primary care, because of the strong association between certain high-risk lifestyles and health care usage, we must have an explicit policy that those people who refuse to adopt healthier lifestyles risk surrendering claims for boundless medical resources paid by third parties. In fact, devoting huge sums of resources to those people who refuse to alter risky behavior and who are noncompliant to medical advice is unethical in light of limited resources at the plan and state levels. This shift in thinking, however, also requires an intensified social responsibility for health education, counseling, and provision of treatment facilities to individuals at risk as well as heightened efforts to reduce social and economic inequalities that produce unhealthy behavior patterns.

Fourth, we must strengthen efforts to rigorously assess all new medical technologies *before* they become widely diffused and put the burden of proof on the purveyors of them. The tendency to rush each new application to market and deal with the consequences later in the end serves society poorly, even if a few individuals might benefit in the short run. All medical innovations should be assessed not only as to safety and efficacy, but also as to their contribution to health outcomes. We believe public policy has imposed a new duty of setting up a system to judge the cost-benefit of medical technology.

Fifth, we need to shift emphasis within health care from curative, episodic medicine to education, health promotion, and disease prevention and to primary care services available to all citizens. To this end, the imbalance between generalists and specialists must be resolved.

Sixth, we must broaden the definition of health care to encompass social and economic factors and thus downplay the current emphasis on medical care. This in turn necessitates confronting the issue of whether continued investments in medical care represent the best use of societal resource for improvement in length and quality of life for the population. In an even broader sense, we need to consider the question of what priority we should put on health as compared to other social goods. Then and only then can we determine how much and what kind of health we need in order to be, as Callahan terms it, a "humane and decent community of human beings."

Seventh, we must establish a continuing and vigorous dialogue on national goals and the future of the republic. The agenda should include a thorough reevaluation of the impact of unbounded individual rights on solidarity and collective good. It should also address the kinds of issues raised by the first five recommendations stated here. Although it is unrealistic to expect that these basic policy shifts can be accomplished in the short run, because they are so alien to American perceptions of health care, they must become part of the broader debate that to this point has obscured them. If some or all are rejected, so be it, but at least they should be deliberated. Citizens must be given all the facts as to the course we are on.

In order to accomplish these goals, society must set limits through some form of global budgeting to control the amount of resources devoted to medical care. Global budgeting of both public and private spending will also allow restructuring the incentive structure to aid in shifting priority from curative to primary health care. As noted by David Mechanic, managed competition without global budgeting offers little possibility of slowing dynamic forces that accelerate the costs and application of new technologies. Although a single-payer system is the most effective means to global controls, it is highly implausible in the United States. More attention should be given to a national fee structure of the kind Japan has used quite successfully in controlling costs while providing universal coverage in a largely private insurance system.

It must be emphasized that though other countries are better poised to deal with escalating health care problems, no nation has solved the problem of providing health to their citizens. Moreover, every nation has to live with its history; for example, we have the employer as part of our system and it will be hard to remove. It has been estimated that the move to a single-payer system would require almost a trillion dollars of costs now paid by the employer to be transferred to taxes, certainly a political impossibility. In the end, however, setting limits to health needs and to medical progress will require that constraints be imposed from outside by political compulsion. Every nation, including the United States, has to consider cost control at the state and national level. Either competition, regulation, or some combination of the two must be made to work. Cost controls come in two broad categories, financing controls and reimbursement controls, and though no nation has perfected either of them, none has as bad a track record as the United States in this regard. The lesson learned from abroad is that given the high economic stakes involved, self-regulation by definition will not work. Moreover, the costs of health care are substantially related to the size of the health care infrastructure. Every time we add a doctor, hospital, or piece of medical technology, the cost has to be amortized. Government has a duty to "right size" the system to the extent it can. Only through government imperative is this feasible and the chance of controlling health care costs a possibility.

The need to deliberate the limits of medical care, the individual's responsibility for his or her own health, and the broad health goals of society is urgent, and the debate long overdue. Although these actions call for courageous political leadership, ultimately the government cannot legislate new beliefs or values on these issues, either within the medical profession or the public. But it must take the lead. The illusions held by the public that we do not need rationing and that more medicine leads to better health will not easily be shattered, even with zealous leadership and animated dialogue, because these illusions are comfortable and reassuring, especially for the insured population and the medical industry. People are highly resistant to dispelling these illusions, in part because they serve powerful interests, but also because they allow all of us to avoid a harsh reality that we have been led to believe applies only to other nations. The illusions reinforce our feelings of superiority, of being first. The reality of course is that we are not first, nor on many health measures are we even a distant second. Moreover, the reality of the future of our health care system is far from comforting, although under these illusions many would continue to naively treat health care as business as usual. Many health experts and political leaders know we are on a sure path to disaster, but getting society to understand this is most difficult, because there are many forces working to perpetuate the illusions for their own interests or their own peace of mind. The key to resolving the health care crisis ultimately will turn on whether society as a whole can alter its perspectives and accept the reality of the need for constraints on its expectations of what is medically and economically feasible. Without such a major rethink, no amount of incremental change will make our health care system sustainable into the near future.

References

Aaron, Henry J. "Should Public Policy Seek to Control the Growth of Health Care Spending?" *Health Affairs* (January 8, 2003).

Aaron, Henry J., and William B. Schwartz. "Rationing Health Care: The Choice before Us." *Science* 247:418–422.

Alexander, G. Caleb, Rachel M. Werner, and Peter A. Ubel. "The Costs of Denying Scarcity." *Annals of Internal Medicine* 164 (6): 593–96.

Alexander, G. Caleb, Rachel M. Werner, A. Fagerlin, and Peter A. Ubel. "Public Support for Physician Deception of Insurance Companies." *Archives of Internal Medicine* 138:472–75.

Atkins, David, Joanna Siegel, and Jean Slutsky. "Making Policy When the Evidence Is in Dispute." *Health Affairs* 24 (1): 102–13.

Altman, Drew E. and Larry Levitt. "The Sad History of Health Care Cost Containment as Told in One Chart." *Health Affairs* (January 23, 2002).

Altman, Stuart H., Christopher P. Tompkins, Efrat Eilat, and Mitchell P. V. Glavin. "Escalating Health Care Spending: Is It Desirable or Inevitable?" *Health Affairs* (January 8, 2003).

Baily, Mary Ann. "Managed Care Organizations and the Rationing Problem." *The Hastings Center Report* 33 (1): 34–44.

Baker, Laurence, Howard Birnbaum, Jeffrey Geppert, David Mishol, and Erick Moyneur. "The Relationship between Technology Availability and Health Care Spending." *Health Affairs* (November 5, 2003).

Balko, R. *Curbing Your Enthusiasm.* Washington, D.C.: Cato Institute, 2006.

Banks, James, Michael Marmot, Zoe Oldfield, and James P. Smith. "Disease and Disadvantage in the United States and in England." *Journal of the American Medical Association* 295:2037–45.

Banta, David. "The Development of Health Technology Assessment." *Health Policy* 63 (2): 121–32.

Batavia, Andrew I. "Disability Versus Futility in Rationing Health Care Services: Defining Medical Futility Based on Permanent Unconsciousness—PVS, Coma, and Anencephaly." *Behavioral Sciences and the Law* 20:219–33.

Beauchamp, Dan E. *The Health of the Republic: Epidemics, Medicine, and Moralism as Challenges to Democracy.* Philadelphia: Temple University Press, 1988.

Berk, Marc L., and Alan C. Monheit. "The Concentration of Health Care Expenditures, Revisited." *Health Affairs* 20 (2): 9–18.

Berk, Marc L., Claudia L. Schur, Debbie I. Chang, Erin K. Knight, and Lawrence C. Kleinman. "Americans' Views about the Adequacy of Health Care for Children and the Elderly." *Health Affairs* (September 14, 2004).

Blanchette, Patricia "Age-Based Rationing of Health Care." *Hawaii Medical Journal* 54:507–509.

Blank, Robert H., and Viola Burau. *Comparative Health Policy.* Basingstoke: Palgrave, 2004.

———, and Janna C. Merrick. *End of Life Decision Making.* Cambridge, MA: MIT Press, 2005.

Blendon, Robert J., and John M. Benson. *Public Opinion Update on Health Care Reform.* Boston: Harvard Program on Public Opinion and Health Care, 1994.

Blustein, Jan, and Theodore R. Marmor. "Cutting Waste by Making Rules: Promises, Pitfalls, and Realistic Prospects." *University of Pennsylvania Law Review* 140 (5): 1543–72.

Bodenheimer, Thomas. "High and Rising Health Care Costs. Part 1: Seeking an Explanation." *Annals of Internal Medicine* 142 (10): 847–54.

———. "High and Rising Health Care Costs. Part 2: Technologic Innovation." *Annals of Internal Medicine* 142 (11): 932–37.

———. "High and Rising Health Care Costs. Part 3: The Role of Health Care Providers." *Annals of Internal Medicine* 142 (12): 996–1002.

———, and Alicia Fernandez. "High and Rising Health Care Costs. Part 4: Can Costs Be Controlled While Preserving Quality?" *Annals of Internal Medicine* 143 (1): 26–31.

Bohs, Tom. "Coming Soon to an Insurance Plan Near You: Health Care Rationing." *The Jackson (TN) Sun*, April 11, 2004.

Brock, Dan W. "Justice, Health Care, and the Elderly." *Philosophy and Public Affairs* 18:297–312.

———. "Broadening the Bioethics Agenda." *Kennedy Institute of Ethics Journal* 10 (1): 21–38.

———, and Norman Daniels. "Ethical Foundations of the Clinton Administration's Proposed Health Care System." *Journal of the American Medical Association* 27:1189–96.

Brook, Robert H. "The Health Care Resource Allocation Debate: Defining Our Terms." *Journal of the American Medical Association* 266 (1991): 3328–31.

Buchanan, Allan. "Managed Care: Rationing without Justice, But Not Unjustly." *Journal of Health Politics, Policy, and Law* 23 (4): 687-95.

Budetti, Peter P. "10 Years beyond the Health Security Act Failure: Subsequent Developments and Persistent Problems." *Journal of the American Medical Association* 292 (16): 2000–06.

Butter, Irene H. "Premature Adoption and Routinization of Medical Technology: Illustrations from Childbirth Technology." *Journal of Social Issues* 49 (2): 11–34.

Califano, Joseph A. Jr. "Rationing Health Care: The Unnecessary Solution." *University of Pennsylvania Law Review* 140 (5): 1525–38.

Callahan, Daniel. *Setting Limits: Medical Goals in an Aging Society.* New York: Simon and Schuster, 1987.

———. "Symbols, Rationality, and Justice: Rationing Health Care." *American Journal of Law and Medicine* 18 (1–2): 1–13.

———. *False Hopes: Why America's Quest for Perfect Health Is a Recipe for Failure.* New York: Simon & Schuster, 1998.

Center for the Evaluative Clinical Sciences. "The Care of Patients with Severe Chronic Illness: An Online Report on the Medicare Program." *The Dartmouth Atlas of Health Care* 2006, http://www.dartmouth atlas.com.

Chadwick, Ruth. "Justice in Priority Setting." In *Rationing in Action*. London: BMJ Publishing Group, 1993, pp. 85–95.

Churchill, Larry. *Rationing Health Care in America: Perceptions and Principles of Justice*. Notre Dame, Indiana: Notre Dame University Press, 1987.

———. *Self-Interest and Universal Health Care: Why Well-Insured Americans Should Support Coverage for Everyone*. Cambridge: Harvard University Press, 1994.

Clinical Advisory Board. "Elevating the Standard of Critical Care," 2001.

Clinton, William. "U.S. Must Strengthen and Fix Health Care System." From President's Address on Health Care. September 22, 1993.

Coast, J., et al. "If There Were a War Tomorrow, We'd Find the Money: Contrasting Perspectives on the Rationing of Health Care." *Social Science and Medicine* 54:1839–51.

"Cost Burdens Influencing the Delivery of Intensive Care: The Growing Strain on Resources Contributes to

Rationing of Medical Care for Critically Ill Patients." *Critical Care Nursing Quarterly* 26 (4): 335–39.

Cundiff, David, and Mary Ellen McCarthy. *The Right Medicine: How to Make Health Care Reform Work Today.* Totowa, NJ: Humana Press, 1994.

Daniels, Norman. *Am I My Parents' Keeper? An Essay on Justice Between the Young and the Old.* New York: Oxford University Press, 1988.

———. "Justice, Health and Healthcare." *American Journal of Bioethics* 1:2–16.

———, and J. E. Sabine. *Setting Limits Fairly: Can We Learn to Share Medical Resources?* New York: Oxford University Press, 2002.

Davis, Karen. "Consumer-Directed Health Care: Will It Improve Health System Performance?" *HSR: Health Services Research* 39 (4): 1219–33.

Dey, I., and N. Fraser. "Age-Based Rationing in the Allocation of Health Care." *Journal of Aging and Health* 12 (4): 511–37.

Dobson, Roger. "Report Urges More Honest Approach to Rationing." *British Medical Journal* 322:316.

———. "Older People in Queues for Surgery Might Make Way for Younger People." *British Medical Journal* 324:1544.

Doyal, L. "Public Participation and the Moral Quality of Healthcare Rationing." *Quality in Healthcare* 7:98–102.

Duncan, Emily. "U.S. Health Care Is Dismal and Inefficient." Technician via *U-Wire* (January 13, 2005).

Eddy, David M. "What Do We Know About Costs?" *Journal of the American Medical Association* 244:1161–66.

———. "What Care Is 'Essential'? What Services Are 'Basic'?" *Journal of the American Medical Association* 265 (6): 782–88.

———. "Rationing Resources While Improving Quality." *Journal of the American Medical Association* 272 (10): 817–24.

Elhauge, Einer. "Allocating Health Care Morally." *California Law Review* 82 (6): 1449–1544.

Ellner, Andrew. "Rethinking Prescribing in the United States." *British Medical Journal* 327:1397–1400.

Emanuel, Ezekiel J., and Linda L. Emanuel. "The Economics of Dying: The Illusion of Cost Savings at the End of Life." *New England Journal of Medicine* 330 (8): 540–44.

Engelhardt, H. Tristram, Jr. "Allocating Scarce Medical Resources and the Viability of Organ Transplantation." *New England Journal of Medicine* 311 (1): 66–71.

Enthoven, A. "Is There Convergence between Britain and the United States in the Organisation of Health Services?" *British Medical Journal* 310 (6995): 1652–55.

Finkelstein, Eric A., Ian C. Fiebelkorn, and Guijing Wang. "National Medical Spending Attributable to Overweight and Obesity: How Much, and Who's Paying?" *Health Affairs* (May 14, 2003).

Fisher, E. S., John E. Wennberg, Therese A. Stukel, D. J. Gottlieb, F. L. Lewis and E. L. Pinder. "The Implications of Regional Variations in Medicare Spending. Part 2: Health Outcomes and Satisfaction with Care." *Annals of Internal Medicine* 138 (4): 288–98.

Fitzgerald, Faith T. "The Tyranny of Health." *New England Journal of Medicine* 331 (3): 196–98.

Fleck, Leonard M. "Rationing: Don't Give Up: It's Not Only Necessary, but Possible, if the Public Can Be Educated." *The Hastings Center Report* 32 (2): 35–38.

Floyd, Elizabeth J. "Health Care Reform through Rationing." *Medical Benefits* 20 (17): 9–10.

Foster, David. "Frequent Flyer Racks up Big Bill." *Denver News*, October 10, 2001.

Fox, Maggie. "Medicare to Cover Viagra under New Drug Benefit." *Reuters* (February 1, 2005).

Fox, Renee. *The Sociology of Medicine: A Participant Observer View*, 1992, p. 224.

Freeman V., S. Rathore, K. Weinfurt, K. Schulman, and D. Sulmasy. "Lying for Patients: Physician Deception of Third-Party Payers." *Archives of Internal Medicine* 159:2263–70.

Friedenberg, R. "Health Care Rationing: Every Physician's Dilemma." *Radiology* 217:626–28.

Fries, James F. "Aging, Illness, and Health Policy: Implications of the Compression of Morbidity." *Perspectives in Biology and Medicine* 31:408–32.

Fuchs, Victor. "What Every Philosopher Should Know about Health Economics." *Health Economics* 140:186–95.

———. "Reflections on the Socio-Economic Correlates of Health." *Journal of Health Economics* 23 (4): 653-61.

Fuller, Benjamin F. *American Health Care: Rebirth or Suicide?* Springfield, IL: Charles C. Thomas, Publisher, 1994.

Gaylin, Will. "Faulty Diagnosis." *Harper's Magazine* (October 1993).

Giacomini, M. "The Which Hunt: Assembling Health Technologies for Assessment and Rationing." *Journal of Health Politics, Policy and Law* 24:715–58.

Ginsburg, Marjorie E. "Perspective: Cost-Effectiveness: Will the Public Buy It or Balk?" *Health Affairs* (May 19, 2004).

Ginsberg, Eli. "High-Tech Medicine and Rising Health Care Costs." *Journal of the American Medical Association* 263 (13): 1820–22.

———. "The Uncertain Future of Managed Care." *New England Journal of Medicine* 340:144–46.

Goodman, M. "Ethical Issues in Health Care Rationing." *Nursing Management* 5:29–33.

Goodman, John C. "To Your Health: Commentary." *Wall Street Journal*, December 26, 2003, p. A10.

Graig, Laurine A. *Health of Nations: An International Perspective on U.S. Health Care Reform*, 2nd ed. Washington, D.C.: Congressional Quarterly Press, 1993.

Hadorn, David C., and Robert H. Brook. "The Health Care Resource Allocation Debate." *Journal of the American Medical Association* 266 (23): 3328–31.

Hall, M. "The Public's Preference for Bedside Rationing." *Archives of Internal Medicine* 156:1353.

———. *Making Medical Spending Decisions: The Law, Ethics, and Economics of Rationing Mechanisms*. New York: Oxford University Press, 1997.

Ham, Chris, and A. Coulter. "Explicit and Implicit Rationing: Taking Responsibility and Avoiding Blame for Health Care Choices." *Journal of Health Sciences and Research Policy* 6 (3): 163–69.

Havighurst, C. C. "Prospective Self-Denial: Can Consumers Contract Today to Accept Health Care Rationing Tomorrow?" *University of Pennsylvania Law Review* 140 (5): 1555–1608.

Heffler, Stephen, Sheila Smith, Sean Keehan, M. Kent Clemens, Mark Zezza, and Christopher Truffer. "Health Spending Projections through 2013." *Health Affairs* (February 11, 2004).

Herper, Matthew. "Cancer's Cost Crisis." *Forbes* (June 8, 2004).

Hiatt, Howard. "Protecting the Medical Commons." *New England Journal of Medicine* 293 (5): 235–41.

Hope, Tony. "Rationing and Life-Saving Treatments: Should Identifiable Patients Have Higher Priority?" *Journal of Medical Ethics* 27:179–185.

———, Nicholas Hicks, D. J. M. Reynolds, Roger Crisp, Sian Griffiths. "Rationing and the Health Authority." *British Medical Journal* 317:1067–69.

Illich, Ivan. *Limits to Medicine: Medical Nemesis: The Expropriation of Health.* London: Penguin Books, 1976.

Jeffrey, S., J. Groeger, K. Kalpalatha, et al. "Descriptive Analysis of Critical Care Units in the United States: Patient Characteristics and Intensive Care Unit Utilization." *Critical Care Medicine* 21(2): 279–91.

Josefson, Deborah. "Gatekeeping May Not Be Cost Effective." *British Medical Journal* 323:1090.

Kapp, Marshall. "De Facto Health-Care Rationing by Age." *Journal of Legal Medicine*, 19:323–49.

Kassler, Jeanne. *Bitter Medicine: Greed and Chaos in American Health Care*. New York: Birch Lane Press, 1994.

Keenan, Patricia S. "What's Driving Health Care Costs?" Issue Brief, *Commonwealth Fund* (November 2004).

Kitzhaber, John. "A Healthier Approach to Health Care." In Robert H. Blank and Andrea L. Bonnicksen, eds., *Emerging Issues in Biomedical Policy,* Vol. 1. New York: Columbia University Press, 1992.

Klein, Rudolf. "Why Britain Is Reorganizing its National Health Service—Yet Again?" *Health Affairs* 17 (4): 111–25.

Lasser, Karen E., David U. Himmelstein, and Steffie Woolhandler. "Access to Care, Health Status, and Health Disparities in the United States and Canada: Results of a Cross-National Population-Based Survey." *American Journal of Public Health* 96 (7): 1300–1307.

Leichter, Howard M. *Free to be Foolish: Politics and Health Promotion in the United States and Great Britain.* Princeton: Princeton University Press, 1991.

Lenaghan, J. "Involving the Public in Rationing Decisions." *Health Policy* 49:45–61.

Levit K., et al. "Trends in U.S. Health Care Spending, 2001." *Health Affairs* 22:154–64.

Lewins, Frank W. *Bioethics for Health Professionals.* New York: Macmillan, 1996.

Light, Paul. *The Politics of Social Security Reform.* New York: Random House, 1985.

Lomas, J., and A. P. Contandriopoulos. "Regulating Limits to Medicine: Towards Harmony in Public- and Self-Regulation." In Theodore R. Marmor, ed., *Understanding Health Care Reforms.* New Haven: Yale University Press, 1994, pp. 253–286.

Marchione, Marilynn. "Doctors Say Futile Cancer Treatment Rising." *AP*, June 12, 2006.

Marmor, Theodore R., and David Boyum. "American Medical Care Reform: Are We Doomed to Fail?" In Theodore R. Marmor, ed., *Understanding Health Care Reform.* New Haven: Yale University Press, 1994.

Marmot, Michael, and Richard G. Wilkinson, eds. *Social Determinants of Health.* Oxford: Oxford University Press, 1999.

Maynard, Alan. "Ethical Issues in the Economics of Rationing Healthcare." *British Journal of Urology* 76:59–64.

———. "Rationing Health Care: An Exploration." *Health Policy* 49:5–11.

———. "Ethics and Health Care 'Underfunding.'" *Journal of Medical Ethics* 27:223–27.

Mechanic, David. "Professional Judgment and the Rationing of Medical Care." *University of Pennsylvania Law Review* 140:1713–54.

———. *Inescapable Decisions: The Imperatives of Health Care.* New Brunswick, NJ: Transaction Publishers, 1994.

———. "Muddling through Elegantly: Finding the Proper Balance in Rationing." *Health Affairs* 16:83–92.

Melcer, Rachel. "U.S. Must Limit Access to Health Care, Experts Say." *St. Louis Post-Dispatch*, October 8, 2004, p. N4.

Menzel, Paul T. "Some Ethical Costs of Rationing." *Law, Medicine and Health Care* 20 (1): 57-66.

Minkler, M. "Personal Responsibility for Health: A Review of the Arguments and the Evidence at Century's End." *Health Education and Behavior* 26 (1): 121–40.

Mokdad, A. H., J. S. Marks, D. F. Stroup, and J. L. Gerberding. "Actual Causes of Death in the United States." *Journal of the American Medical Association* 291:1238–45.

Monheit, Alan C. "Persistence in Health Expenditures in the Short Run: Prevalence and Consequences." *Medical Care* 41 (7): III53–III64.

Morgall, Janine Marie. *Technology Assessment: A Feminist Perspective.* Philadelphia: Temple University Press, 1993.

Morreim, E. Haavi. "Gaming the System: Dodging the Rules, Ruling the Dodgers." *Archives of Internal Medicine* 151:443–47.

———. "Moral Justice and Legal Justice in Managed Care: The Ascent of Contributive Justice." *Journal of Law, Medicine and Ethics* 23:247–65.

Mullen, P. "Rational Rationing?" *Health Services Management Research* 11:113–23.

Nicklaus, David. "Health Care Problem? Actually, U.S. Has Two." *St. Louis Post-Dispatch*, September 26, 2004.

Office of Technology Assessment. *Development of Medical Technology: Opportunities for Assessment.* Washington, DC: GPO, 1976.

———. *Strategies for Medical Technology Assessment.* Washington, DC: GPO, 1982.

Olshansky, S. Jay, Bruce A. Carnes, and Christine Cassel. "In Search of Methuselah: Estimating the Upper Limits of Human Longevity." *Science* 250:634–40.

Orentlicher, D. "Practice Guidelines: A Limited Role in Resolving Rationing Decisions." *Journal of the American Geriatrics Society* 46:369–72.

Pauly, Mark V. "Should We Be Worried about High Real Medical Spending Growth in the United States?" *Health Affairs* (January 8, 2003).

Perneger, T., et al. "Physicians' Attitudes toward Health Care Rationing." *Medical Decision Making* 22:65-70.

Morgall, Janine Marie. *Technology Assessment: A Feminist Perspective.* Philadelphia: Temple University Press, 1993.

Perry, Seymour. "Medical Technology in a Cost Containment Environment." In *The Future of Health in America.* Hearings before the Joint Economic Committee, United States Congress, May 1988. Washington, D.C.: GPO, 1989.

PricewaterhouseCoopers. *Cost of Caring: Key Drivers of Growth in Spending on Hospital Care* (February 19, 2003).

Pulskamp, John R., Bradley G. Williams, and Hugh G. Walsh. "HMOs Broke the Golden Mandate." *Wall Street Journal,* October, 20, 1999, p. A27.

Rai, A. "Rationing through Choice: A New Approach to Cost-Effectiveness Analysis in Health Care." *Indiana Law Journal* 72:1014–97.

Regalado, Antonio. "Rationing Health Care in an Age of Rising Costs." *Wall Street Journal*, 2004.

Relman, Arnold S. "The Trouble with Rationing." *New England Journal of Medicine* 323 (13): 911–13.

Rill, Jonathan. "Universal Care Means Rationing." *St. Louis Post-Dispatch*, May 30, 2004, p. A15.

Rivlin, M. "Can Age-Based Rationing of Health Care be Morally Justified?" *The Mount Sinai Journal of Medicine* 64:113–19.

Rogers, A., et al. "If a Patient Is Too Costly They Tend to Get Rid of You: The Impact of People's Perceptions of Rationing on the Use of Primary Care." *Health Care Analysis* 7:225–37.

Roos, Noralou P., Evelyn Shapiro, and Robert Tate. "Does a Small Minority of Elderly Account for a Majority of Health Care Expenditures? A Sixteen-Year Perspective." *Milbank Quarterly* 67 (3/4): 347–69.

Rosen, Rebecca, and John Gabbay. "Linking Health Technology Assessment to Practice." *British Medical Journal* 319:1292.

Rosenbaum, David E. "What If There Is No Cure for Health Care's Ills?" *The New York Times*, September 10, 2000.

Rosenthal, Meredith, and Arnold Milstein. "Awakening Consumer Stewardship of Health Benefits: Prevalence and Differentiation of New Health Plan Models." *Health Services Research* 39 (4 Pt 2): 1055–70.

Russell, Barbara J. "Health-Care Rationing: Critical Features, Ordinary Language, and Meaning." *Journal of Law, Medicine and Ethics* 30 (1): 82–89.

Saint Louis Post-Dispatch. "U.S. Health Care: A Sick System: How Other Nations Do It." January, 3, 2005, p. NA.

Savage, David G., and Alissa J. Rubin. "High Court Sides with HMOs in Suit over Cost-Cutting." *Los Angeles Times*, January 13, 2000.

Schur, Claudia L., Marc L. Berk, and Jill M. Yegian. "Public Perceptions of Cost Containment Strategies: Mixed Signals for Managed Care." *Health Affairs* (November 10, 2004).

Schwartz, William B., and Daniel N. Mendelson. "Eliminating Waste and Efficiency Can Do Little to Contain Costs." *Health Affairs* 13 (2): 224–38.

Scitovsky, Anne A. "The High Cost of Dying: What Do the Data Show?" *Milbank Memorial Fund Quarterly* 62:591–607.

Scott, Jeanne S. "Dare We Use the Word (Gasp)—'Rationing'?" *Healthcare Financial Management* 58 (5): 32–34.

Shaw, A. "Age as a Basis for Healthcare Rationing." *Drugs and Aging* 9:403–6.

Sher, George. "Health Care and the 'Deserving Poor.'" *Hastings Center Report* 13(2): 9–12.

Shortt, Janet. "Obesity—A Public Health Dilemma." *AORN Journal* 80 (6): 1069–1076, 1078.

Singer, Peter A. "Medical Ethics." *British Medical Journal* 321:282–85.

———. "A Strategy to Improve Priority Setting in Health Care Institutions." *Behavioral Science and Medicine* 11(1): 59–68.

Singer, Peter A., Douglas K Martin, Mita Giacomini, Laura Purdy. "Priority Setting for New Technologies in Medicine: Qualitative Case Study." *British Medical Journal* 321:1316–18.

Skinner, Jonathan S., Douglas O. Staiger, and Elliott S. Fisher. "Is Technological Change in Medicine Always Worth It? The Case of Myocardial Infarction." *Health Affairs* (February 7, 2006): W34–W47.

Smith, G. "Our Hearts Were Once Young and Gay: Health Care Rationing and the Elderly." *University of Florida Journal of Law and Public Policy* 8:1–23.

———. "Allocating Health Care Resources to the Elderly." *Elder Law Review* 1:21–27.

Stevens, Andrew, and Ruairidh Milne. "Keeping Pace with New Technologies: Systems Needed to Identify and Evaluate Them." *British Medical Journal* 319:1291.

Stukel, Therese A., F. Lee Lucas, and David E. Wennberg. "Long-Term Outcomes of Regional Variations in Intensity of Invasive vs. Medical Management of Medicare Patients with Acute Myocardial Infarction." *Journal of the American Medical Association* 293: 1329–37.

Sullivan, Louis W. "Healthy People 2000." *New England Journal of Medicine* 323:1065–67.

Tanner, Lindsey. "U.S. Newborn Survival Rate Ranks Low." *AP*, May 5, 2006.

Tauber, Alfred I. "Medicine, Public Health, and the Ethics of Rationing." *Perspectives in Biology and Medicine* 45 (1): 16–30.

———. "A Philosophical Approach to Rationing." *MJA* 178 (9): 454–56.

Thorpe, Kenneth E., Curtis S. Florence, and Peter Joski. "Which Medical Conditions Account for the Rise in Health Care Spending?" *Health Affairs* (August 25, 2004).

———. Curtis S. Florence, David H. Howard, and Peter Joski. "The Impact of Obesity on Rising Medical Spending." *Health Affairs* (October 20, 2004).

Ubel, Peter A. *Pricing Life: Why It's Time for Health Care Rationing.* Cambridge: MIT Press, 2000.

———. "Time for Physicians to Take the Lead in Health Care Rationing." *Geriatric Times* (September 1, 2003): 30.

———, and R. Arnold. "The Unbearable Rightness of Bedside Rationing." *Archives of Internal Medicine* 155:1837–42.

———, and S. D. Goold. "Rationing Health Care: Not All Definitions Are Created Equal." *Archives of Internal Medicine* 158 (3): 209–14.

Vandewater, Judith. "Healing the U.S. Health System: There's No Easy Cure." *St. Louis Post-Dispatch*, October, 17, 2004, p. A1.

Varmus, Harold. In *What Price Better Health?: Hazard of the Research Imperative* by Daniel Callahan. Berkeley: University of California Press, 2006.

Veatch, Robert M. "Allocating Health Resources Ethically." *Frontiers of Health Services Management* 8 (1): 3–29, 43–44.

Weale, Albert. "Rationing Health Care." *British Medical Journal* 316:410–26.

Weinstein, Milton C. "Should Physicians Be Gatekeepers of Medical Resources?" *Journal of Medical Ethics* 27:268–74.

————. "We Ration Health Care: Better to Do It Rationally." *The Washington Post*, June, 1, 2003, p. B3.

Wennberg, John E., Elliott S. Fisher, Laurence Baker, Sandra M. Sharp, and Kristen K. Bronner. "Evaluating the Efficiency of California Providers in Caring for Patients with Chronic Illnesses." *Health Affairs* (November 16, 2005) 10.1377/hlthaff.w5.526.

Werner, R. M., G. C. Alexander, A. Fagerlin, and P. Ubel. "The 'Hasstle Factor': What Motivates Physicians to Manipulate Reimbursement Rules?" *Archives of Internal Medicine* 162:1134–39.

"Who Gets What in Critical Care? Task Force Tackles Care Rationing Initiative to Yield Ethical Guidelines for Limiting Treatment." *Critical Care Alert* 11 (8): 95–96.

Williams, B. O. "Ageism Helps to Ration Medical Treatment." *Health Bulletin* 58 (3): 198–202.

Williams, A. "Rationing Health Care by Age: The Case For." *British Medical Journal* 314:820–22.

Yamey, Gavin. "Health Secretary Admits that NHS Rationing Is Government Policy." *British Medical Journal* 320:10.

Yoder, Stuart. "Individual Responsibility for Health: Decision, Not Discovery." *Hastings Center Report* 32 (2): 22–31